A Parent's Guide to
CYSTIC FIBROSIS

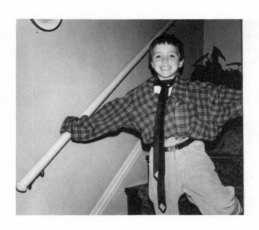

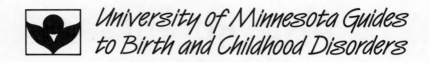

University of Minnesota Guides to Birth and Childhood Disorders

Edited by Robert J. Gorlin
Regents Professor of Oral Pathology and Genetics,
and Professor of Pediatrics, University of Minnesota

Subjects of Forthcoming Volumes

Cerebral palsy	Leukemia	Spine deformities
Kidney disorders	Sickle-cell anemia and thalassemia	

A Parent's Guide to

CYSTIC FIBROSIS

Burton L. Shapiro, Ph.D., professor of oral science and laboratory medicine and pathology, and member of the Institute of Human Genetics at the University of Minnesota Health Science Center

and

Ralph C. Heussner, Jr., medical writer, University of Minnesota

University of Minnesota Press
Minnesota   Oxford

Published by the University of Minnesota Press
2037 University Avenue Southeast, Minneapolis, MN 55414
Printed in the United States of America on acid-free paper

Library of Congress Cataloging-in-Publication Data

Shapiro, Burton L.
    A parent's guide to cystic fibrosis / Burton L. Shapiro and Ralph
C. Heussner, Jr.
        p.   cm. — (University of Minnesota guides to birth and
childhood disorders)
    Includes bibliographical references.
    Includes index.
    ISBN 0-8166-1488-1 (hc). — ISBN 0-8166-1490-3 (pb)
    1. Cystic fibrosis in children—Popular works.   I. Heussner,
Ralph C.   II. Title.   III. Series.
    [DNLM: 1. Cystic Fibrosis—popular works.   WI 820 S529p]
RJ456.C9S45   1990
618.92'37—dc20
DNLM/DLC
for Library of Congress   90-11033
                                                                    CIP

A CIP catalog record for this book is available from the British Library

The University of Minnesota
is an equal-opportunity
educator and employer.

CONTENTS

FOREWORD

A Parent's Guide to Cystic Fibrosis is a volume in a series addressing the needs not only of parents but also of physicians and persons concerned with the care of children with relatively common disorders. We used as a model *The Child with Down's Syndrome*, written by David W. Smith, M.D., and Ann Asper Wilson, first published in 1973 by W. B. Saunders, Philadelphia. The book is very valuable because it makes the complex concepts of genetics and pediatrics understandable to parents. Such is the goal of our series.

In *A Parent's Guide to Cystic Fibrosis*, it was the authors' intent to provide parents and other health-care givers with a knowledgeable discussion of the nature and cause of cystic fibrosis together with genetic risks, the clinical picture, vignettes from one family, how the disorder affects the body, how the diagnosis is made, current modes of therapy, complications, psychosocial aspects, social resources, and, finally, the molecular detection of the carrier state and prenatal detection of this most important single-gene recessive disorder. If one considers that in some populations, 1 in 20 individuals is a carrier and that about 70% of these mutations can be detected, the sheer task of identifying those who wish "to know" is prodigious.

The book was written by Burton L. Shapiro, M.S., Ph.D., and Ralph C. Heussner, Jr. Burton Shapiro is presently professor in the Department of Oral Sciences and in the Department of Laboratory Medicine and Pathology at the University of Minnesota, Minneapolis, Minnesota. He earned an M.S. in Oral Pathology and a Ph.D. in Genetics at the University of Minnesota. Dr. Shapiro has devoted most of his research career to pursuing the mechanisms involved in the pathogenesis of cystic fibrosis. Studying the metabolism of connective tissue cells from patients with cystic fibrosis, he was the first to report markedly elevated intracellular calcium levels and increased oxygen consumption by both affected individuals and carriers of the disease. Ralph Heussner is currently medical writer and editor for the Department of Laboratory Medicine and Pathology and study coordinator for the AIDS Clinical Trials Unit at the University of Minnesota. I first became acquainted with Ralph Heussner after reading the superb *Herpes Diseases and Your Health*, which he wrote with Henry H. Balfour, Jr., M.D., published by the University of Minnesota Press in 1984. The combined effort of Burt Shapiro and Ralph Heussner in writing *A Parent's Guide to Cystic Fibrosis* is indeed a most fortunate amalgam.

The need for this series is obvious. Parents with a child who has a serious disability need answers. They need to know not only the nature of their child's disorder but also its possible causes, its prognosis, the limitations it will impose on the child, the impact it will have on the entire family, and the chances of it recurring in either the parents' future children or in the affected child's children. It is also important that parents be informed about community resources that can help them deal with the disorder. And, certainly, they need to know what they themselves can do to help.

In spite of good intentions, the health professional has not always been an effective communicator. These books are designed to open the lines of communication between the health professional and parents by increasing parents' understanding and providing them with a basic vocabulary for easier and more accurate expression of the worries, doubts, and uncertainties attendant on each disorder. It is our intention that health professionals play a vital role in supplementing each text with their own expertise. We cannot hope to answer all the questions that may be posed by parents, but we believe that each book will go a long way in answering many of the common ones.

R.J.G.

PREFACE

"The most common life-threatening genetic disease of Caucasian children."

No doubt, every parent of a child with cystic fibrosis will have heard that statement by the time he or she reads this book.

Though true, the sentence is too general to give valuable insight into the problem. It presumes that all children with cystic fibrosis will follow the same course. They do not. To some people, the term "genetic" often implies that medical intervention cannot alter the course of the disease. But it can!

The fact that you are reading this book means that you want to have a better understanding of cystic fibrosis. You are still searching for answers to questions that may be practical ("Should my child receive routine immunization shots?") or philosophical ("Why did this happen to my child?").

We do not yet fully understand cystic fibrosis. Although the scientific puzzle is slowly coming together, many pieces are still missing. Nevertheless, medical science has made significant steps to improve and extend the lives of individuals with cystic fibrosis.

Our purpose in writing this book was to explain the genetic causes and biological effects of the disease as well as its social and psychological aspects. We describe how the body's various systems—respiratory, digestive, reproductive, and musculoskeletal—respond to cystic fibrosis. We discuss the rationale behind some of the strategies used to keep the disease under control. We address recent advances in treatment and outline some of the horizons of research that may prove helpful to your child in the future.

As you know, parents play a pivotal role in the care of children with cystic fibrosis. Therefore, we have personalized our story with comments from parents and patients throughout the text, a separate chapter devoted to Family Life, and selections from a "family diary" at the end of chapters 1-6. Please remember in reading this diary that it represents one patient's experience. The procedures recommended for this boy may not be appropriate for all children with cystic fibrosis. In addition, because of ever-improving treatment, some of the therapies described may no longer be in use at the time you read this book.

We have attempted to put a complex disease into a context and language that is complete, yet understandable. To help you comprehend what may seem like the foreign language of genetics and medicine, we have included an extensive glossary at the back of the book. For parents who desire additional information, a list of resources is provided.

Becoming more knowledgeable about the disease will help you:

—Understand the genetic causes and biological effects of cystic fibrosis.

—Appreciate the need for the aggressive daily care required to keep symptoms of cystic fibrosis under control.

—Communicate better with your doctors and, as a result, enable you to make more intelligent decisions about treatments for your child.

—Prepare to deal with the psychosocial ramifications of cystic fibrosis.

—Provide a basis for understanding new treatments or research developments as they are certain to unfold in the years ahead.

Please keep in mind as you read this book that every child is unique and there is neither a "typical" disease course nor a universally effective management and treatment plan. About the only constant is what you—mother or father—choose to give your child in terms of love, kindness, support, and understanding.

For years, cystic fibrosis was considered, almost exclusively, an early childhood disease because so few survived beyond childhood. That has changed dramatically. Because of great strides made in recent decades in the understanding and treatment of the disease, the average age reached by those with cystic fibrosis continues to climb. It has become not just a disease of children, but a disease of adults, as well.

We wish to thank Jim Winterer for providing the Family Diary sections, which are based on his family's personal experiences.

A Parent's
Guide to
CYSTIC
FIBROSIS

Chapter 1
THE GENETIC BLUEPRINT

"*It's not fair and someone must be wrong. They told me that if Bob and I are both carriers of cystic fibrosis, the chances are only one-in-four that we would have a baby with the disease. Well, three of our four kids have cystic fibrosis. That can't be right. Most other families have only one kid with it.*"

A young couple decides to have a child. They are both healthy and, as far as they know, no major genetic disease has occurred in either family. After a smooth pregnancy, a baby boy is born. He sleeps well and has a superb appetite, but there is some delay in regaining his birth weight. After he has several bouts with colds and is not able to gain weight despite hearty eating, the baby's doctor orders a sweat test.

"Your baby has cystic fibrosis," says the doctor, reading from a laboratory report. Gently, calmly, the doctor tells the parents about the disease and its complicatons—respiratory infections and digestive disorders. The doctor describes the type of treatment the child will have, emphasizing how the health of children with cystic fibrosis has improved significantly in recent years.

The doctor advises the young couple that they are both genetic carriers of this disease.

"How could that be," they wonder? "Both of us are healthy. No relative on either side of the family has ever had cystic fibrosis. How could our baby have a genetic defect? And if the doctor is right, why are our other children healthy?"

To answer these and other questions, we must begin with a discussion of cells, chromosomes, and genes. Consider this chapter a short course in human genetics. Understanding the principles of heredity may help you resolve some of your questions about how and why cystic fibrosis occurred in your son or daughter.

What Are Genes and Chromosomes?

Let's begin by looking through the microscope at a single cell of the body. As we increase the magnification of the microscope, we can detect the various parts of the cell, including its nucleus, the center of the cell. If we look closely, we can detect tiny threadlike bodies in the nucleus. They're called chromosomes (Figure 1).

Each chromosome is composed of two materials: proteins and deoxyribonucleic acid (DNA). DNA carries the information of heredity in discrete units called genes. Think of a chromosome, then, as a string of genes similar to a necklace of pearls.

Genes control heredity, passing on the blueprint of life from parents to children. They instruct cells to manufacture special proteins, such as those that form hair, or to divide so that the organism will grow or so that a wound will heal.

Most human body cells each have 23 pairs or a total of 46 chromosomes—23 from the mother's ovum or egg and 23 from the father's sperm—thought to contain between 50,000 and 100,000 genes. In 1985 after decades of research, three independent groups of scientists proved that the cystic fibrosis gene resides on chromosome 7. It is fairly certain that nearly everyone who is affected by cystic fibrosis has the

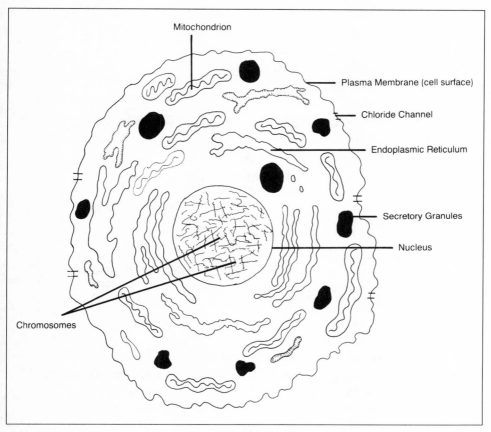

FIGURE 1

An idealized cell. Information for all cell functions is stored in the nucleus on chromosomes. Each chromosome carries hundreds or thousands of genes, depending on its size. Blueprints for manufacturing proteins that end up in secretory granules pass from the nucleus to the endoplasmic reticulum where proteins are made. Energy for all cell functions is generated in mitochondria. Small molecules, such as chloride and water, move through channels in the cell membrane. More elaborate systems permit secretion of large molecules in secretory granules from the cell.

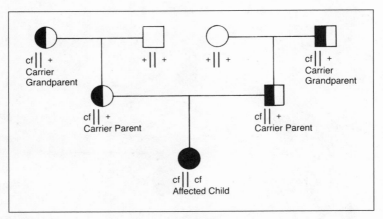

FIGURE 2
A pedigree of a family with cystic fibrosis. ○ = female and □ = male. A
completely filled symbol represents person (in this case, female) with cystic
fibrosis. Half-filled symbols are healthy carriers for cystic fibrosis. Beneath
each symbol is shown two number 7 chromosomes. Both chromosomes in
the affected child (one from each of her parents) have information for the
cystic fibrosis protein. Each of the carriers has one copy of the cystic fibrosis
gene and one copy of the normal counterpart.

same abnormal gene. (It is known now that the precise gene
abnormality may be different in different families.)

Tracing Your Family Tree

When discussing genetics, your physician or a genetic counselor usually begins by drawing a diagram of a family tree,
also called a pedigree (see Figure 2). As you see, both parents
contributed a cystic fibrosis gene to their affected child, and
both sets of grandparents passed the cystic fibrosis genes to
these parents.

Your child has received a "double dose" of the gene that
codes for cystic fibrosis. Geneticists refer to conditions that
require this double dose of an abnormal gene as a "reces-

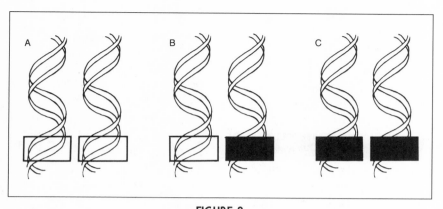

FIGURE 3
A diagram of a portion of chromosome 7. ☐ = genetic information for
the normal gene at the cystic fibrosis site; ■■ = the cystic fibrosis gene. A =
a person normal for the cystic fibrosis gene; B = a healthy carrier for cystic
fibrosis; C = an individual with a double dose of the cystic fibrosis gene,
hence affected.

sive" trait. (When a single abnormal gene is sufficient to
have an effect, the trait caused by that gene is called "dominant.") Cystic fibrosis cannot be passed on by one parent
alone. The product of a recessive gene is suppressed when it
is matched with its normal counterpart. Only one gene and
its protein product are necessary for normal function. Such is
the case in parents of children with cystic fibrosis. They each
have one dose of the normal protein, even in the presence of
an abnormal counterpart, and that is sufficient for normal
functioning. But if both forms of this gene are abnormal, the
clinical problems associated with cystic fibrosis arise.

If an individual possesses the normal information in both
chromosomes of this pair, he or she is normal for this gene
(Figure 3A). If an individual has one chromosome with the
normal information and one with the cystic fibrosis variant,
the person is functionally normal because a single normal
gene is sufficient for normal functioning (Figure 3B). A third
possibility is an individual who has the cystic fibrosis gene
on both chromosomes (Figure 3C). This individual has no

cellular genetic information for manufacturing the normal gene product needed by many glands and, hence, is affected by cystic fibrosis.

Both parents are healthy because a single dose of the abnormal gene does not cause any problems. They are called "carriers" of the abnormal gene. About 10 million individuals in the United States, 2 million in Great Britain, and 1 million in Canada are carriers of the gene responsible for cystic fibrosis. Less than 1% realize they carry the gene; they discover it only when an affected child is diagnosed. The Cystic Fibrosis Foundation estimates that approximately 30,000 people in the United States, 6,500 in Great Britain, and 3,000 in Canada have cystic fibrosis. It is one of the most common recessive genetic diseases, occurring most frequently among Caucasian populations, especially those of Central and Western European descent.

You may wonder why the severity of cystic fibrosis varies widely from case to case, even in the same family. Some patients have relatively mild symptoms for years or decades with the clinical problems not occurring until adulthood, while others face severe problems from infancy. These differences result from the other thousands of genes in each cell and from environmental conditions (e.g., nutrition, benign life situations, amount of exercise, etc.) that differ for every individual.

The Genetic Risks

What is the risk of acquiring the cystic fibrosis gene?

At each ovulation in a female carrier, an egg will possess the cystic fibrosis gene or the normal gene. Half the sperm produced by a carrier father will possess the cystic fibrosis gene and half will possess the normal gene. Therefore, at each conception there is a one-in-four chance that a child of two carrier parents will have cystic fibrosis, a two-in-four chance that the child will be a clinically normal carrier as is

Table 1. Risks of Having a Child with Cystic Fibrosis		
One Parent	*Other Parent*	*Chances Child Will Have CF*
Known carrier	Known carrier	1 in 4
Known carrier	General population	1 in 80
CF	General population	1 in 40
Sibling of CF	General population	1 in 120
Sibling of CF	Sibling of CF	1 in 9
Aunt or uncle of CF	General population	1 in 160
First cousin of CF	General population	1 in 320
General population	General population	1 in 1,600

each parent and a one-in-four chance that the child will have two normal genes and cannot pass on the cystic fibrosis gene.

It's possible that two carrier parents will never have a child with cystic fibrosis (three-in-four chance at each conception) and will never know that they are carriers. On the other hand (and here's the answer to the parent quoted as the beginning of this chapter), since the one-in-four chance recurs at each conception, carrier parents risk having a child with cystic fibrosis at every conception even though the chances are one-in-four each time.

Table 1 shows the probabilities of producing a child with cystic fibrosis, depending on what is known about the parents. About 1 in 1,600 newborns has cystic fibrosis and about 1 in 20 individuals in the general white population is a healthy, unaffected carrier of cystic fibrosis. The numbers in the table are simply "toss of the coin" odds and are not based on actual statistical studies of occurrence rates. Recently developed techniques of DNA analysis can be applied as early as two months following conception using prenatal diagnosis to give more precise predictions in families where both parents are known carriers. We discuss this technique in more detail on page 81 in Chapter 7, Horizons of Research.

Parents whose first child is affected by a recessive disorder often misunderstand the "risk ratio." They misconstrue the 25% chance or "one-in-four" odds to mean that the next three offspring are not endangered. This is not the case; the risk remains the same for every future child of the same mother and father, in the same way that the odds of coming up with heads in a coin toss is 50% with each toss.

Genetic Counseling

When parents learn that their child has cystic fibrosis and that cystic fibrosis is a genetic disease, they might seek consultation with a genetic counselor. Genetic counselors can explain the origin and consequences of the disorder, as well as the chances that it will recur in another child. For a disorder such as cystic fibrosis that is known to have a single gene inheritance, the recurrence risk for specific family members can be readily determined most of the time.

The genetic counselor's primary role is to provide a factual understanding of the genetic problem. Sometimes the counselor's answers will help to resolve or prevent troubling family situations, such as quarreling or blaming. If parents have suppressed anger or resentment, the counselor may make it possible for those emotions to be expressed.

When the genetic disorder involves recessive inheritance such as cystic fibrosis, normal parents sometimes consider themselves abnormal or defective. The counselor will reassure them that this is not true. Indeed, all of us carry some harmful genes in our biological makeup; it's simply bad luck when both parents carry the same abnormal gene and produce a child with the disease.

Finally, the genetic counselor can explain modern diagnostic techniques. When both parents are known carriers, prenatal diagnosis may be an option they will want to consider. Because it is more likely that an unborn child of two carrier parents will be normal, these tests can relieve parents' anxiety.

The information provided by a genetic counselor can play a positive role psychologically. Psychologists are nearly unanimous in believing that education makes it easier to live with any kind of physical impairment. Also, the background information specifically helps parents to understand treatment options.

Genetic counselors are usually affiliated with major hospitals or University-affiliated medical centers. Your physician can usually arrange for a referral to a licensed counselor.

* * *

In the first installment of our Family Diary, we'll see how one family learned to accept and cope with cystic fibrosis in their son Ben. In subsequent chapters, we'll follow Ben and his parents through some of their unique family experiences associated with the illness. We hope these personal accounts will illuminate the medical discussion in the following chapters.

FAMILY DIARY

Getting Acquainted with Cystic Fibrosis

We sat down in the hospital lobby, stunned and anxious, prepared for a long talk with the doctor about our baby, Ben. Only the day before, a "sweat test" had confirmed the doctor's suspicions: cystic fibrosis was the reason our newborn was so hungry, yet remained terribly thin.

"It's not an easy disease to have—not for the patient or the family," he said. "Sometimes it will be exhausting—physically, emotionally, and financially. But how you deal with it can make a very real difference in the quality of life for your son, and for you, too."

He was right, and it's what doctors ought to tell every family new to cystic fibrosis.

Emotionally, there's a lot to sort out in those first weeks following diagnosis of cystic fibrosis. And there's a lot to learn, too, because most care of young patients takes place at home, not in the hospital.

In some diseases, there's little the family can do. For the most part, care is in the hands of health professionals while parents remain at the bedside, or pace the hallway. But with cystic fibrosis, the roles are reversed. Mothers, fathers, sisters, and brothers all get involved.

And that means, in a matter of weeks, unsuspecting parents become respiratory therapists, pharmacists, insurance whizzes, nutritionists, medical-equipment technicians, social workers, and skilled orators who can explain why kids never outgrow cystic fibrosis, or why such a healthy-looking third-grader takes digestive enzyme pills every time he eats at the local burger joint.

Much of that education, at least in our family, came during Ben's first two-week visit to the university hospital. I'll never forget the first night they draped a clear plastic tent over his crib and turned on the mist machine (a therapy rarely, if ever, used today). As we watched, the surreal fog thickened, and our little wisp of a baby disappeared. I couldn't help but wonder if we'd lose him, and not just in some cloud. He was only six weeks old, and he was dying, fast.

Not many years ago, Ben would have died. The doctors would have said he "failed to thrive." Some might have blamed it on "consumption."

But Ben would benefit from the incredible strides made against cystic fibrosis in the past 30 years. He was lucky to be in one of the nation's leading cystic fibrosis care centers.

Within a few days, Ben turned the corner, thanks to the digestive enzymes. For the first time in his young life, he began to gain weight. What a joy to see chubby cheeks again!

The nurses poked his skinny fingers no end, taking blood samples to determine what other medications he would need. There were plenty—a regular shopping list of enzymes, inhalation solutions, vitamins, and antibiotics.

Therapists taught us to administer bronchodilators to help open Ben's airways, then how to pound his chest, back, and sides to knock it loose. They were hard to please: "No, don't

pound there, that's his heart . . . you forgot that position . . .
don't just pound, cup your hand and make a clop-clop sound
. . . pound faster . . . pound harder, he won't break . . . no,
now you're pounding way too hard."

It wasn't that we resented what was happening. After all,
the drugs and therapy were saving Ben's life. But we were
awed. The sense of responsibility every parent feels at the
birth of a child is one thing, but this seemed overwhelming. So
much to remember. What if we forgot something? What if we
got the drugs mixed up? What about insurance? What about
all these new machines to bring home? What was our life going to be like now?

The answers would come later. Something that helped was
seeing the other babies and their parents on the hospital
ward. Ben was the only CFer in the crowd, and when we
looked around, cystic fibrosis didn't seem so bad. Many of the
babies would never leave the ward. One was brain dead,
others had major deformities. Many would never talk, walk,
or run.

Soon, we'd be going home with our thriving son. We were
the lucky ones.

Chapter 2
HOW CYSTIC FIBROSIS AFFECTS THE BODY

"*It just doesn't make sense. How can one abnormal gene cause Jennie to cough and have fatty stools and salty sweat? And how come some of the other kids with CF don't have fatty stools and still others don't cough. I just don't understand!*"

The symptoms of cystic fibrosis and the severity of these symptoms vary considerably from patient to patient. Indeed, diagnosing cystic fibrosis may be difficult. Although most patients experience pulmonary and/or gastrointestinal problems early in life, their symptoms may be mild. A few may go undiagnosed for years or decades before their chronic symptoms are recognized as cystic fibrosis. Signs of cystic fibrosis in older patients may be male infertility or cirrhosis of the liver.

The characteristics of cystic fibrosis are sometimes mistakenly thought to be chronic bronchitis, pneumonia, asthma, or one of the other conditions associated with the body's inability to properly process food. Not all of the possible characteristics of cystic fibrosis occur in every patient.

If a physician suspects that a child has cystic fibrosis, a "sweat test" will be ordered. This test is a simple, inexpensive, and noninvasive method of diagnosing cystic fibrosis (Figure 4). If it is analyzed in a qualified laboratory, it is extremely accurate. Basically, the test measures the amount of salt in human sweat; an increase in the concentration of

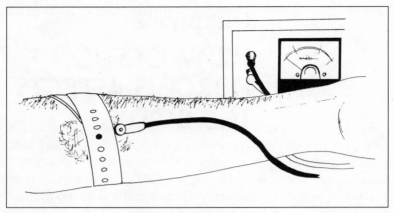

FIGURE 4
Sweat testing. A mild (and safe) chemical that induces sweating is "driven" into sweat glands by a very slight electrical current. After a few minutes, the electrodes are removed and an absorbent material is placed over the same area. Sweat is collected for 30 to 60 minutes and analyzed in the laboratory for chloride or sodium. In the presence of lung or digestive problems very high sweat salt indicates cystic fibrosis.

salt in the presence of lung and/or digestive system abnormalities or a family history of cystic fibrosis indicates cystic fibrosis.

Most patients will experience the common symptoms of cystic fibrosis as children. Signs of respiratory distress are chronic bronchitis and pneumonia; difficulty digesting food and presence of fatty stools indicate problems in the gastrointestinal system.

Progressive pulmonary infection is the single most important clinical problem in CF. The leading cause of death is respiratory problems leading to heart failure.

The history of cystic fibrosis has changed dramatically in a relatively short time. In 1971 only 11.3% of patients registered at Cystic Fibrosis Treatment Centers in the United States were over 18 years of age. Today that figure has climbed to almost 30%. Advances in the care of children with cystic fibrosis seem even more significant when viewed historically. To appreciate these improvements, let's briefly trace the history of the disease.

A Brief History of Cystic Fibrosis

Cystic fibrosis is not a new disease. Although it was not defined as a distinct disease entity until the 1930s, many references to children with a "salty taste" and fatty stools can be found as early as the 1600s. In 1705 a German author wrote in a book of folk philosophy that infants who tasted salty were bewitched. The *Almanac of Children's Songs and Games* from Switzerland published in 1857 observed that "the child will soon die whose brow tastes salty when kissed."

One of the earliest medical descriptions of what appears to be cystic fibrosis was published in an autopsy report in 1838. By the early 1900s, numerous articles began to appear describing newborns with pancreatic disorders. Looking back, it appears these disorders were related to cystic fibrosis.

In the 1930s, scientists began to describe cystic fibrosis as a distinct entity, meaning that the symptoms observed were the result of cystic fibrosis and were not related to another illness. The term "cystic fibrosis of the pancreas" was first used by D. H. Andersen in 1938 in a comprehensive description of the disease in 49 patients. After observations of the "new disease," a tremendous amount of research followed as scientists and physicians defined in more detail how cystic fibrosis affects different organs of the body.

In 1944 scientists noted how a widespread defect in mucous secretions could explain many symptoms of cystic fibrosis. The recessive inheritance pattern was proposed in 1946. Major advances in the 1950s involved diagnosis, especially development of the sweat test, and successful treatment of lung infections with antibiotics. In 1985 three independent groups of scientists proved that the defective gene was located on chromosome 7, and late in 1989 the gene itself was characterized (see p. 84).

The Cystic Fibrosis Foundation (CFF), founded in 1955 by a small group of parents and families of patients with cystic fibrosis, has played an integral role in facilitating much of this recent research. Today the foundation includes more than 200,000 volunteers working in more than 70 chapters. In addition to raising funds for basic biomedical and clinical research, the CFF conducts patient service programs, promotes public education, and supports a network of approximately 120 care centers throughout the United States.

Cystic fibrosis affects nearly every organ of the body in either a primary or secondary way. By primary, we mean that the disease impairs the normal functioning of the organ. A secondary effect relates to complications of the disease.

Except for the sweat and salivary glands, cystic fibrosis affects organs in a similar way—abnormal secretions obstruct ducts or tubes. We'll discuss this in more detail later in this chapter.

One of the most important discoveries in cystic fibrosis was that the disease disrupts the normal functioning of exocrine glands. Unlike endocrine glands, such as thyroid, adrenal, and pancreatic insulin-producing glands, which secrete their products internally, exocrine glands secrete their products onto body surfaces or into body cavities. Exocrine glands are found throughout the body and include the pancreas (the non-insulin-producing portions), and the salivary, mammary, tear, and sweat glands. Some single, mucous-secreting cells that line the respiratory and gastrointestinal tracts are also considered part of the exocrine system because their products enter body secretions.

For a general idea of the architecture of exocrine glands, think of a tree with its trunk, main branches, slender branches, and tiny twigs. It's at the tips of the gland's smallest segments that the protein synthesizing portions (acini) empty their products into little tubes or ducts. Small ducts join into larger ones and, like the branches of the tree, connect into even larger ducts. Eventually, the ducts flow into a major tube exiting onto a body surface.

The body has two general types of exocrine glands: some produce watery secretions, such as sweat and tears; others excrete thick and sticky products, such as the respiratory mucus of the nose and lungs. Some glands, such as those that produce sweat, are individually tiny, while others are organized into large major organs, such as the liver and pancreas.

Secretions in the lung in cystic fibrosis are often thick and sticky, causing obstructions in the small airway passages and providing a breeding ground for bacteria (see Chapter 3, The Respiratory System). Pancreatic secretions are especially important in cystic fibrosis because this organ produces important digestive enzymes that break down food so it can be absorbed and metabolized (see Chapter 4, The Gastrointestinal System). These digestive enzymes may be produced in insufficient quantities in cystic fibrosis.

Figure 5 shows a generalized diagram of an exocrine gland. The cells of the bowl-shaped acinus are specialized for the production and delivery of large proteins and protein/sugar molecules into the branched, tree-like tubular systems. (The types of products produced by the acinus vary from gland to gland.) As the secretion passes from the acinus through ducts and tubes of increasing diameter toward the body surface, small molecules are reabsorbed back into the body through the ductal cells. This reabsorption helps prevent the body's loss of important small molecules—such as sodium, chloride, and glucose—through exocrine secretions onto the skin, gut, and respiratory tracts.

Two major biological processes go awry in cystic fibrosis. First, normal portions of these glands may be replaced by scar tissue. As a result, the gland stops working as it should and creates problems in the pancreas and the lungs. Second, some exocrine cells have difficulty transporting salts from secretions back into the body, as is the case in the sweat glands.

To understand how the scarring and destruction occurs in the pancreas and lungs, think again of the tree-like structure of these glands, with the acini at the very tips of the twigs. It is believed that the earliest biological changes caused by cystic fibrosis are micro-obstructions caused by thick and sticky

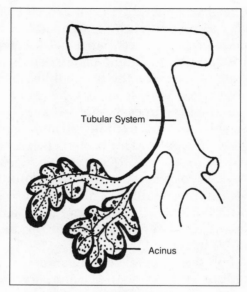

FIGURE 5

A segment of an exocrine gland. Large proteins, many of which are enzymes, are manufactured in clusters of cells called acini. These products enter the tubular and ductal system for transport to body surfaces.

secretions of these acini. The acini secrete their products into plugged connecting tubes. The plugged acini and tubes in cystic fibrosis destroy the acinar cells and balloon their ducts. The ballooning results in swollen ducts, the "cysts." The destroyed tissue is replaced by scar tissue, called "fibrosis."

In the lung, this destructive scarring and ballooning process affects tissues that specialize in the exchange of carbon dioxide waste products from the body with oxygen from the air. Adding to respiratory difficulties is the accumulation of obstructing mucus that, in turn, provides sites for bacterial growth. Medical treatment is aimed at controlling infection and clearing the respiratory plugs.

In the pancreas, similar obstructive changes occur, although infection is unusual. The primary result of pancreatic plugging is loss of cells that usually provide enzymes necessary to break down food in the intestine into smaller molecules to be passed through the gut wall and into the body. For most people with cystic fibrosis, these changes in the pancreas lead to reduced delivery of digestive enzymes to the gut. This, then, leads to malnutrition because foods cannot be digested and are excreted, unused, by the body. Supplemental enzymes—one of the real breakthroughs in treatment of cystic fibrosis—can help patients digest their food.

Sweat glands, another major exocrine tissue dramatically affected by the disease, show no structural changes, even when cells are viewed with a powerful electron microscope. Nevertheless, the cells function abnormally. Small molecules, such as salt, are not reabsorbed normally back into the body. The excessive loss of salt that results gives a salty taste to the skin. It's this level of salt, measured in a "sweat test," that confirms the diagnosis of cystic fibrosis.

How are these seemingly unrelated processes linked? Scientists speculate that a possible common denominator is abnormal cell membrane channels through which salt molecules enter and exit cells. The relationship between this abnormality and the signs and symptoms of cystic fibrosis is not yet understood.

* * *

In the next three chapters, we will discuss in detail the major body systems disturbed by cystic fibrosis. But first let's turn to our Family Diary to see how one family reacted to a diagnosis of cystic fibrosis.

FAMILY DIARY

The Diagnosis

Every "CF parent" can recall that moment when he or she learned for certain their youngster had the disease. It ranks right up there with life's other major memories: the kids' first day of school, the first stitches, the big part in the Christmas pageant, those first wobbly moments without training wheels, and high-school graduation.

It's like someone had just handed you a heavy weight and said, "Here, now carry THAT around for a few years." You feel a swirl of emotions—heartache and confusion, fear and anger, pity and love. The diagnosis of cystic fibrosis can bring a sense of relief, or it can make you feel like the victim of a cruel rip-off. How parents respond to this emotionally wrenching news is determined, at least in part, by their general outlook on life. You can either retreat or move ahead. Is the disease a curse or a challenge?

Early symptoms of cystic fibrosis are similar to those found in more common, yet less severe illnesses. Parents and doctors might first suspect the baby is having trouble shaking a bad cold. The ongoing diarrhea or frequent slimy stools are blamed on a particular strong strain of stomach flu. So parents put up with a runny nose and slimy diapers. But when your child doesn't improve, you begin to worry. Some parents jump from doctor to doctor, trying medication after medication. In desperation, a few turn to quack remedies.

But you don't cure cystic fibrosis with clear broth or cough syrup. And too often children with cystic fibrosis go through several misdiagnoses before the real culprit is finally nailed down. So how would you feel? Here you thought your child just had a runny nose. Big deal. All of a sudden, you've swapped a box of tissues for the nation's number-one genetic killer of children. Maybe you were becoming a little tired of smelly green diapers every hour or so, but now you learn your baby has only a 50-50 chance of living as long as it takes most other kids to finish college and get started on their careers and families. Those irritations and inconveniences now seem so minor, even trivial.

You feel that you and your child have been terribly cheated.

In our family, the diagnosis of Ben's cystic fibrosis brought more relief than anything. He was a beautiful, chubby baby, weighing a hefty eight pounds at birth. But he soon developed a runny nose and a bit of cough. That didn't worry us as much as his weight. He nursed and nursed, but gained no weight. We later learned why: because the tiny ducts that deliver digestive enzymes to his intestine were plugged with sticky mucus, his mother's nutritious milk didn't do him any good. He was literally starving to death and we didn't have a clue why!

Cystic fibrosis symptoms can vary widely from child to child. Ben had a classic case of un-digestion. In a matter of weeks, he had become a quiet, little bag of bones.

Living at the time in a fairly remote area of the state, we were incredibly lucky to have a doctor who suspected, when Ben was about five weeks old, that cystic fibrosis might be the culprit.

Our "country doctor" made arrangements at a university hospital for the standard "sweat test." I remember that day so clearly. We had decided that his mother would take Ben on the 100-mile trip to the hospital while I stayed home with our other child. It was a long spring afternoon, waiting and wondering and hoping. I was puttering out in the yard when I finally heard the car pull up. Nothing had to be said. I knew, from the look in his mother's eyes, that Ben had the disease.

But now Ben also had a chance. Without the correct diagnosis, medications and treatments, he wouldn't have lived much longer. Now the fight was on, and we were happy for it.

Chapter 3
THE RESPIRATORY SYSTEM

"**E**very fall at the start of school, our daughter's new teacher would tell us that Karen was sick. The teacher would say that Karen's constant cough was disruptive and probably spreading germs throughout the class. 'Take her to a doctor!' the teacher would say. Karen has probably seen more doctors than all the kids in the class put together."

To understand lung problems in cystic fibrosis you first need to understand how the lungs work normally. All activities of living organisms are fueled by energy, and one of the ingredients needed to create this energy is oxygen. The process of converting oxygen into a biologically useful form is called oxidation.

Since only small amounts of oxygen can be stored in the body, an uninterrupted supply of oxygen to each cell is necessary to maintain metabolism. We use the term "respiration" to refer to those processes by which cells use oxygen, produce carbon dioxide, and convert energy to biologically useful forms. The respiratory system consists of the lungs and the tubes through which air reaches them (Figure 6).

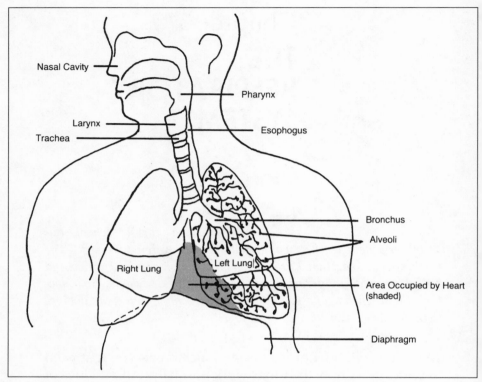

FIGURE 6

The respiratory system. Air passes through the nose and mouth through a system of tubes—the trachea, bronchi, and bronchioles—to air sacs (alveoli). At the site of the air sacs, oxygen passes into the blood system for circulation throughout the body. Carbon dioxide formed from respiration in body cells passes from the blood system into air sacs for expiration.

Normal Functioning of the Lungs

Respiratory function consists of two processes: ventilation and respiratory gas exchange. Ventilation is the movement of air into the spaces where the exchange of gases takes place (alveolar spaces). In respiratory gas exchange, oxygen and carbon dioxide move across tiny, thin-walled air sacs into

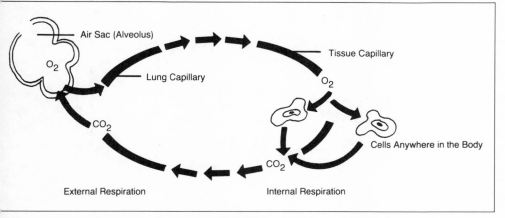

FIGURE 7

Respiration. In the lung, oxygen from inhaled air passes from air sacs into tiny blood capillaries, and carbon dioxide passes from the capillaries into air sacs. Throughout the body oxygen passes from capillaries into cells for energy while carbon dioxide passes from the cells into capillaries for removal from the lungs.

(and out of) capillaries (Figure 7), tiny thin-walled blood vessels that connect arteries and veins. Arteries circulate oxygen throughout the body, and veins return carbon dioxide to the lungs for expiration. The presence of fluid, scar tissue, or infection between the membranes of the capillaries and of the lung hampers the exchange of gases, thus causing disease.

The lungs begin to form early in the development of the fetus. They start as hollow, tubular outgrowths of simple tubes in the embryo, growing into the "respiratory system" that ultimately includes the nose, mouth, pharynx, larynx, trachea, bronchus, lungs, and the intricate network of tubes throughout the lungs (Figure 6).

Call to mind, once again, how exocrine glands are shaped like trees. Let's follow the process of air through the system. Air enters the body through the nose and mouth and passes through the pharynx and larynx to the trachea. The trachea branches into two large bronchi, major tubes (or branches)

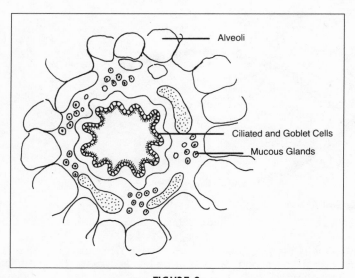

FIGURE 8
Normal small bronchus. Lined by ciliated and goblet (mucous) cells. Compare with Figure 10.

that enter the right and left lung. The bronchi branch into smaller bronchioles which, in turn, branch repeatedly into small tubes ultimately leading to tiny air sacs. In the walls of air sacs are minute, cup-shaped cavities, the alveoli, which are associated with a rich network of capillaries. This is where the exchange of oxygen and carbon dioxide occurs. It is estimated that the surface area of these alveoli is more than 50 times the area of the skin.

All but the smallest branches of the respiratory tree are lined with ciliated (hairlike structures) epithelial cells (cells that cover internal and external surfaces of the body and that make up a major portion of organs) heavily mixed with mucus-secreting cells (Figure 8). The mucus and cilia have important functions. The mucus moistens the air we breathe and prevents drying of delicate alveolar walls. Bacteria, dust, and other small particles are trapped by the mucus. The hairlike cilia, meanwhile, beat constantly in one direction

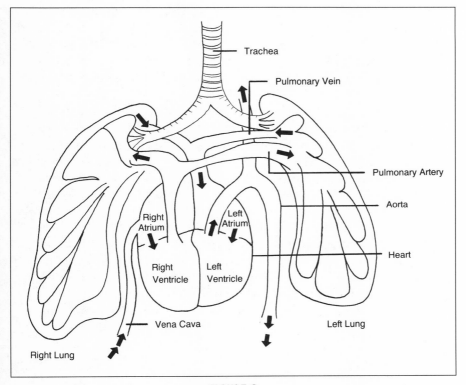

FIGURE 9

Circulation of blood through the heart and lungs. The heart has four chambers and valves, which prevent backflow of blood. Blood containing freshly inhaled air moves from the lungs through the pulmonary veins to the left atrium and then to the left ventrical where it is pumped into arteries for transport throughout the body. After giving up oxygen to cells and now containing carbon dioxide produced during metabolism, blood moves back to the heart through veins. The blood enters the right atrium through the large vena cava. It is pumped into the right ventricle and from there back to the lungs by way of the pulmonary arteries. Lung disease can cause the right ventricle to overwork and may lead to its enlargement.

and aid in removing of foreign material and contaminated mucus by propelling it back into the large bronchi and trachea. Once there, our cough reflex finishes the task of expelling contaminated or foreign materials. This ciliary action is important, since the upright posture of humans favors downward drainage of foreign material, fluid, and debris into the deepest parts of the lungs. Numerous glands are located throughout the walls of the trachea, bronchi, and bronchioles that contribute mucous secretions to the respiratory tubes.

Oxygen passes from alveoli to pulmonary capillaries while carbon dioxide flows in the reverse direction. The pulmonary artery brings blood to the lung by way of the heart from areas throughout the body (Figure 9). This blood contains carbon dioxide generated by cell metabolism of glucose and other substances. The carbon dioxide in the pulmonary capillaries is at a higher concentration than in air breathed in, and it diffuses out of the blood vessels, into the lungs, and is breathed out. Conversely, because the oxygen in a fresh breath of air is at a higher concentration than in blood returning to the lungs from the body, it flows in from the alveoli to the pulmonary capillaries for distribution throughout the body. This respiratory gas exchange depends on the condition of the alveolar membrane and its capacity to permit the interchange of oxygen and carbon dioxide.

A resting adult breathes in and out about half a liter of air (the equivalent of a pint) with every breath. By contracting abdominal muscles, an additional 1.5 liters can be expelled. Still another liter remains in the lung that cannot be expelled. During normal breathing, a reserve of about 2.5 liters of air remains in the lungs and mixes with the half-liter inhaled in an average breath. After a normal breath, it is possible, by inhaling deeply, to take in as much as three liters more.

One method of analyzing your respiratory status is to measure air volume, also known as "vital capacity" of the lungs. Here's how it's done: a person breathes in as deeply as possible, then breathes out as completely as possible into a device called a spirometer that can gauge air volume. This is the maximum volume of air that can be expired slowly and completely after a full breath is taken. Though simple, this test is one of the most valuable measurements of pulmonary function. Older children with cystic fibrosis will have the test re-

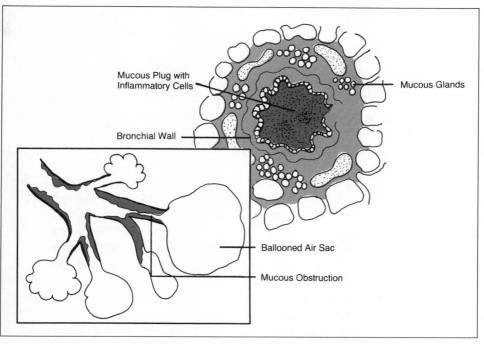

FIGURE 10
Infection and obstruction in a small bronchus in cystic fibrosis. When this figure is compared with Figure 8, you can see an increased number of mucous
glands, loss of cilia on lining cells, and a break of the lining. The inset shows
ballooned air sacs caused by the bronchial obstruction and inflammation.

peated periodically. Results are compared with previous
measurements to determine the child's respiratory condition. More than two dozen additional tests are available to
evaluate pulmonary function.

Common Lung Problems

The phrase "chronic obstructive pulmonary disease"
(COPD) succinctly describes the most serious medical prob-

lem in cystic fibrosis. The lungs' air passages, normal at birth, eventually become plugged. And plugging leads to respiratory distress. Most patients experience chronic coughing, wheezing, and recurring lung infections. Because the lungs of children with cystic fibrosis are structurally normal at birth, infection, inflammation, and environmental pollution would seem to be responsible for development of respiratory problems.

The earliest problem in pulmonary functioning occurs when the small tubes (bronchioles) leading to the air sacs become plugged by mucus and inflamed, a condition known as bronchiolitis. Accompanying early bronchiolitis is a decrease in the ciliated cells, resulting in stickier mucus with fewer cilia available to help carry it away. As the problems compound, bacterial infections may develop in the mucous plugs, and the larger tubes may become inflamed (chronic bronchitis) and plugged. This may be accompanied by a ballooning and weakening of the bronchial wall (bronchiectasis) and a resulting infection (Figure 10).

Chronic infection by germs (or, in medical parlance, pathogens) is a major pulmonary problem. Early in the disease, the bacteria *Staphylococcus aureus* are most frequently found in lungs. As the disease progresses, *Pseudomonas aeruginosa* becomes the most frequent germ afflicting patients. Once established, these bacteria are extremely difficult to get rid of. The increased mucus, decreased ciliary action, and resulting infection generate a cycle of more obstruction. The large airways become filled with sticky products of the lungs and of the bacteria. Multiple small abscesses (pneumonia) may occur throughout the lung. To prescribe the appropriate antibiotic, the physician must identify the germ responsible for the infection.

Management of respiratory problems is designed to combat and reverse the "cycle of obstruction" as early as possible. If the lung problems progress despite treatment, respiratory and/or heart failure can result. In respiratory failure, the exchange of gases between the circulating blood and the outside air is impaired. This decreased delivery of oxygen and removal of carbon dioxide affect cellular metabolism in organs throughout the body.

Obstruction and scarring of the lungs affect the right ventricle of the heart, which pumps blood to the lungs. Lung obstructions force the heart to work harder, often leading to enlargement of this chamber. Ultimately, the heart may be unable to circulate blood.

Treatment of Lung Problems

Of the many symptoms and complications of cystic fibrosis, lung problems are the most serious and the most difficult to treat. Despite major advances in treatment, respiratory failure remains the leading cause of the signs and symptoms of the illness and of death. Routine treatment of pulmonary problems typically includes a two-pronged approach: daily clearing of sticky mucus from the lungs, and the use of antibiotics to fight germs. Early and aggressive treatment of lung problems is one of the keys to successful long-term management of cystic fibrosis.

A common method for clearing the respiratory passages is chest physiotherapy — "pounding" — to produce bronchial or postural drainage, that is, forced drainage of mucus from deep in the lungs to be coughed up or spit out. As we discussed earlier, mucus is normally cleared by ciliary movement, breathing out of air, coughing, and swallowing. Because the respiratory fluids in cystic fibrosis are too thick to flow freely, they must be cleared out. The daily routine of rigorous "pounding" of your child's chest makes up for the body's inefficiency (Figure 11).

During each bronchial drainage treatment, the patient is positioned and rotated so that the bronchial tubes are drained downward. A respiratory therapist will demonstrate the proper technique of pounding. After several minutes of vigorous clapping of the chest, the area is vibrated with the hands as the patient deeply exhales. As secretions move into

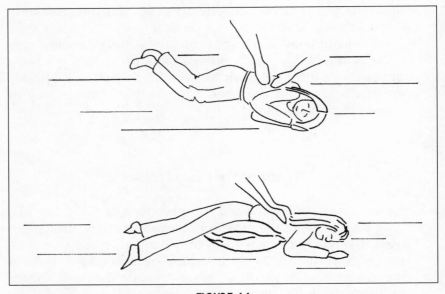

FIGURE 11

Postural drainage. Two of the approximately dozen positions used to remove mucus from areas in the lungs.

larger tubes, the patient is encouraged to cough. The coughing reflex helps clear the lungs. All lobes must be drained daily. In some patients, the treatment must be repeated several times a day.

Several mechanical devices allow patients to perform their own chest physiotherapy. This is beneficial because it allows the individual to be less dependent on parents and other caregivers. It is especially important to adolescents and young adults.

In some cases, bronchodilators (drugs that expand the tubes of the lungs) or mucolytics (substances that thin the mucus) are administered by aerosol before the bronchial drainage clapping. Oral expectorants and mist tents, common techniques in the past, are no longer routinely used. Coughing is the most effective way for the body to remove mucus from air passages. Therefore, children should be encouraged to cough during bronchial drainage and at other times. Cough suppressants should not be used because coughing is helpful in clearing the lungs.

"Doug has always been particularly active, just like I was when I was a kid, I guess. When he first started school and the teachers learned he had cystic fibrosis, they kept telling him not to exert himself, to take it easy. I was able to attend a meeting at school of all the teachers and explained about cystic fibrosis and how it's good for him to run and jump and be just as active as possible. Now they tell Doug to push as hard as he can. It's good for him."

Studies have shown that physical activity stimulates coughing and contributes to the overall fitness of your child. In a recent study in Sweden, researchers demonstrated conclusively that a daily program of aggressive physical exercise improved pulmonary function. The study involved 12 patients (6 boys and 6 girls) 14-25 years of age. Physical activity was adjusted to personal interest and capacity, and prescribed twice a day for a minimum of 15 minutes each time. They participated in vigorous programs of sit-ups, rope-jumping, trampolining, jogging, swimming, and ball games. At the end of the study, the researchers suggested that a good program of physical activity was as efficient as conventional chest physiotherapy. They added that the "psychological advantage was great and . . . contributed to a more independent childhood and a better quality of life for these patients." Of course, you should consult with your physician before instituting a formal exercise program for your child.

Improved antibiotics (drugs used to prevent or treat bacterial infections) have dramatically improved the health and prognosis of individuals with cystic fibrosis. Antibiotics are effective against many of the common micro-organisms including *Staphylococcus aureus*, *Hemophilus influenzae*, and *Pseudomonas aeruginosa*. Depending on the case, antibiotic therapy might be periodic or long term. Severe lung infections may require hospitalization for treatment with larger-than-usual doses of antibiotics delivered intravenously (via a tube inserted in an arm vein).

New techniques of antibiotic administration have also contributed to the improved health of cystic fibrosis patients. For example, recent evidence suggests that antibiotics in aerosols may be useful for controlling stubborn *Pseudomonas* infections.

Immunization against respiratory viral diseases such as pertussis (whooping cough), measles, and influenza is routine. Yearly influenza boosters are necessary because the common strains frequently change each winter.

Other Respiratory Problems

Complications of progressive lung disease may include coughing up blood (hemoptysis), which is usually an indication of increased infection, and the accumulation of air between the covering membranes of the lung (pneumothorax). Pneumothorax may lead to a collapsed lung in a few patients. The condition occurs suddenly, usually beginning with a severe sticking pain in the side and great difficulty in breathing.

More than 90% of patients with cystic fibrosis suffer from sinusitis, the inflammation of the linings of the air-filled cavities in head bones that are connected with the nostrils. About 15% have small benign growths, called polyps, in their nasal passages. It is believed that both sinusitis and nasal polyps result from congestion of the mucous membranes lining the nasal passages by abnormally thick secretions. Sinusitis can be treated medically, but polyps may have to be removed surgically.

* * *

In the next installment of our Family Diary, we'll see how Ben and his family fit the daily bronchial drainage regimen into their family schedule, and how they coped with a "near crisis" when Ben scored poorly on a routine respiratory examination.

FAMILY DIARY

Could a Kitten Do All That?

Our golden retriever, one of the mellowest creatures on earth, had lived longer than he had any right to. At age 15, he finally wore out.

But we missed him sleeping underfoot. It was time for another family pet and the kids, Ben and Will, had their hearts set on a cat.

So along came Emily, a tailless Manx. With hind legs longer than her front, she looked and acted—even hopped—like a rabbit.

We had Emily only a few weeks, just long enough for the family to become firmly attached to her. She seemed to be especially fond of me. Fluffy, innocent Emily loved to sink her kitten claws into my big toe while I did Ben's bronchial drainage treatments—a twice-a-day pounding routine most kids with cystic fibrosis go through to knock loose the sticky mucus in their lungs.

Ben had recently turned eight, and it was time for his quarterly checkup at the cystic fibrosis clinic. He seemed in good shape to me, although I noticed some wheezing now and then.

They ran Ben through the routine tests, including pulmonary function tests to check the efficiency and capacity of his lungs. The results were poor; his lungs were out of whack. For kids with cystic fibrosis, that's depressing news. The doctor advised hospitalization, but we talked him into letting Ben return home for a week to see if things improved.

It wasn't a crisis, but it was time to turn up the wick. We increased his medications and intensified home therapy.

Instead of three inhalation treatments of bronchodilator at 10 minutes each, he'd do four at 15 minutes. Instead of two routine bronchial drainage sessions we'd do four. Instead of just pounding his chest with my cupped hands, I'd also haul out the percussor, a vibrating disk that helps jiggle sticky mucus from his lungs.

Two treatments a day fit fairly well into a family routine: one before breakfast, the other before bed. But when the treatments are longer and there are twice as many, cystic fibrosis is no longer routine. It becomes all-consuming. Housework piles up. Laundry is laughed at. Mail is ignored. Bills go unpaid. The only thing that gets cleaned out is the refrigerator. It means getting up before dawn for the first treatment; interrupting work and school schedules for another at noon; squeezing one in before supper; and finally, after the dishes, starting all over again.

You can keep up that routine for a few days, but when it drags on for a week or more, therapy starts taking a toll on your child and on you. One day blurs into the next. I once calculated that I pounded Ben's chest about 13,000 times for the longer treatments—over 50,000 times a day. Your arms never seem to recover, if you're doing it right. And doing it right—a respiratory therapist told me at a recent cystic fibrosis conference—means "you should work up a good sweat by the time you're done."

Meanwhile, everyone's supply of patience goes bankrupt, and even kitten claws tugging at your toe aren't cute anymore. But you keep it up, because everyone is home, and that's better than the hospital.

When the week was up, we returned to the clinic to retake the pulmonary function tests and X-rays. Ben flunked again. After hours and days of extra pounding, his airways were worse than ever.

As the doctor and I sat down for a talk in the examination room, he looked stumped. The tests showed no infection. Ben wasn't losing weight. Although there wasn't much more the hospital could do than we could do at home, it looked like Ben was going to be admitted anyway. The doctor kept flipping through Ben's medical charts, looking for clues. "The lungs aren't infected, he said, "but they're obstructed. It seems like it could be an allergic reaction."

I suddenly remembered Emily. I think it was because my toe hurt. "Did you know we got a cat a few weeks ago?" I volunteered, almost feeling guilty, as if we'd committed a crime. "You've got a what?" the doctor replied, raising an eyebrow. "A cat. This cute little kitten with big back legs and . . ."

"You've got to get rid of it," he said firmly. "Today! This afternoon! Now!"

I knew we weren't going to talk him out of that one. How can you argue with success? Our cystic fibrosis clinic has an outstanding track record for keeping kids with cystic fibrosis healthy.

I felt sorry for the doctor. Who wants to tell a kid to get rid of his new little pet because it was making him sick? I appreciated him giving Ben the news rather than having me do it.

Ben was stoic. In a cracked voice, he said, "Dad, let's go home."

We didn't have to stay in the hospital after all. We drove straight home, picked up Emily, and headed to the Humane Society. I let Ben ride in the back of the truck with the cat. I suppose that wasn't good sense medically, but sometimes a parent has to compromise. If Ben got another dose of cat dander, too bad.

Ben remained in the truck while I took Emily inside the animal shelter. I signed the papers, hoping she'd find another nice toe to attack someday and two kids like Ben and Will to love her.

"Do you want to sit up here on the way home?" I asked Ben while climbing back into the truck.

"Naw. I'll ride back here."

"Okay. Hey, Ben, it's okay to feel sad. I sure do." Sliding shut the window that separates the front seat from the camper area where Ben chose to ride, I jammed a Bruce Springsteen tape into the stereo and cranked it good and loud.

It was time for Ben to be alone. Me too. I punched the seat. "Stupid, stupid disease. It won't even let us have a cat."

We shampooed the carpets and furniture at home, and continued the intensive treatments for three more days before returning to the clinic. The follow-up pulmonary function tests would tell us if Emily had been the problem.

Ben passed the tests with flying colors! He was just fine. It was back to routine treatments again . . . back to the real world. We just had to do it without our furry friend.

Chapter 4
THE DIGESTIVE SYSTEM

"**T**he worst part, I think, was when friends visited and asked if something was wrong with the plumbing. The house really stank. When I told them that the baby had problems digesting her food, they looked at me kind of funny. After the diagnosis, when I added enzymes to Betsy's food, it got a lot better."

All animals require carbohydrates, fats, proteins, vitamins, minerals, and water for cell synthesis and cell maintenance. After food and liquids are swallowed, enzymes break them down. The digestive process is like trying to pass pebbles through a strainer. A large pebble won't go through unless it is pulverized into many small fragments. Digestive enzymes serve the same function as the pebble pulverizer—breaking down complex materials so they can pass through the walls of the digestive tract into the body for use by cells.

Normal Gastrointestinal Function

The digestive system—also called the gastrointestinal system—is basically a continuous tube or tract divided into different segments with distinct structures. Associated glands transport various substances to these segments. The entire system is designed to absorb nutrients into the body and excrete undigested waste material.

Several gastrointestinal disorders are common in cystic fibrosis. The most significant problem occurs in the pancreas, the body's primary source of digestive enzymes.

After food is chewed and swallowed, it passes through the pharynx, esophagus, stomach, small intestine, and large intestine (Figure 12). Food is modified at each stage along the digestive pathway. Products from two major organs—the liver and pancreas—enter the tube at the first portion of the small intestine (also called the duodenum) and contribute to the breakdown and absorption of fats and proteins across the intestinal wall. These products mix with the intestinal contents, breaking them down into digestible size. Bile and bile salts from the liver and its storage sac, the gallbladder, enter the intestine along with pancreatic enzymes.

The pancreas is composed of bundles of acinar cells connected to a series of ducts leading to the intestine (Figure 13). The connection to the intestine began in the developing fetus as a tubular outgrowth from the small intestine. As with the other exocrine glands, the pancreas remains connected—by a tube—to the surface from which it arose. As it develops, the pancreas forms into branches of smaller and still smaller tubes and ducts. Those portions farthest from the intestinal surface, and next to the smallest tubes, develop into acinar cells that synthesize proteins. Intermixed with the exocrine portion of the pancreas are endocrine cells that manufacture insulin for delivery directly into the blood system.

The pancreas is the body's major source of enzymes that break down the proteins, fats, and carbohydrates in foods. After the digestive enzymes have broken down the large molecules of proteins, sugars, and fats, the products are absorbed through the wall of the intestine, especially the small intestine. A decrease in these enzymes into the gut causes one of the major problems in cystic fibrosis.

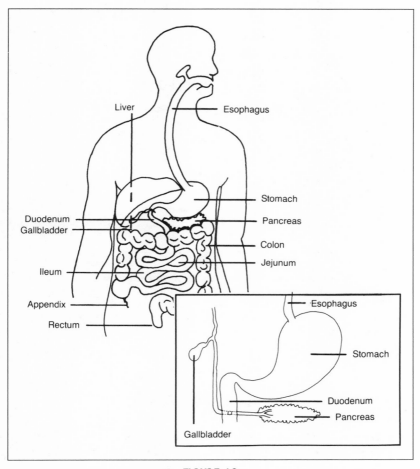

FIGURE 12

The digestive system. Food passes from the mouth through the esophagus to the stomach. At the beginning of the small intestine (duodenum), just after food exits from the stomach, digestive substances enter the small intestine from the pancreas and gall bladder. These substances, most of which are enzymes, are necessary for complete breakdown of foods so that they can cross the intestinal wall to enter the blood system for nourishment of the body.

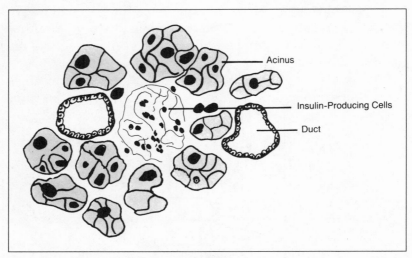

FIGURE 13
A small area of the pancreas as seen through a microscope. Most of the
pancreas is made up of cells (acinar) that manufacture digestive enzymes
which are delivered to the intestine through tubes or ducts. Dispersed
throughout the pancreas are insulin-producing cells whose product enters
the blood system directly.

Problems with the Pancreas

The name "cystic fibrosis" was first used because of changes
in the pancreas. The pancreatic ducts are extremely narrow.
In a pancreas affected by cystic fibrosis, the thick mucous secretions from the cells lining the ducts do not flow smoothly
and they plug the ducts. Plugging creates pressure which
causes the cells of the secreting portions of the pancreas to
shrink and be replaced by scar tissue—the "fibrosis." Plugging also causes the small and large ducts to balloon, or become "cystic."

The result of the scarring and plugging is a marked decrease in the amount of digestive enzymes delivered to the
intestine. Proteins, fats, and, to a lesser degree, carbohy-

drates cannot be broken down into small units. Food passes down the intestine undigested and much less modified than normal. As a result, the body does not receive adequate nutrition. Subsequently, the excreted stools are altered.

About 90% of patients have signs of pancreatic abnormalities, though in highly varying degrees. Pancreatic abnormalities such as the obstruction of small ducts may occur before birth.

What are the signs of pancreatic insufficiency?

—The earliest indication in the newborn might be a delay in or even failure to regain birth weight. Despite a sometimes voracious appetite, weight gain and growth are subnormal.

—The abdomen might bulge. Fat and muscle masses decrease.

—Stools are frequent, bulky, oily, and foul smelling.

Many tests are available to determine the extent of pancreatic problems. These include staining a small stool sample with a dye that stains fat. Very bright staining indicates much fat, a sign of pancreatic insufficiency. Or, stools may be examined directly for reduced amounts or absence of pancreatic digestive enzymes.

The inability to digest food has far-ranging consequences. Besides abnormal stools, the inability to digest fatty substances creates other, more severe problems. For some vitamins to cross the intestinal wall for absorption into the body, they first must be dissolved in and enter with fat. Vitamins A, D, E, and K are fat-soluble, so patients experiencing pancreatic problems may have deficiencies of these vitamins. Poor digestion of protein can lead to protein deficiency, degenerative changes of organs, and the accumulation of fluid in body spaces.

Pancreatic insufficiency in cystic fibrosis has widespread effects. Because changes in the pancreas cannot be treated directly, each consequence must be dealt with individually.

Treatment of Pancreatic Deficiency:
Diet and Nutrition

Pancreatic deficiency is treated mainly by adding enzymes and vitamin supplements to your child's diet. Traditionally, specialized diets for children with cystic fibrosis were designed to be high in calories and proteins and low in fats. However, recent evidence suggests the contrary—food intake is inadequate and getting enough calories is difficult without normal or near-normal fat intake.

Thanks to our new understanding of pancreatic-replacement therapy and the availability of many more effective enzyme supplements, absorption of dietary fat and protein has improved. Dietary restrictions, such as limiting fat intake, have been relaxed, allowing most patients to eat a NORMAL diet.

Dietary changes have promoted nearly normal growth in many children with cystic fibrosis. It's much easier to meet their normal requirements of calories and fatty acids. Nevertheless, intestinal malabsorption remains a serious problem, and diets of children must be monitored closely.

Following diagnosis of pancreatic insufficiency, your child's doctor will probably prescribe pancreatic enzymes that are consumed with every meal and snack. They are extracts from the panceas of hogs that break down fats, proteins, and starches into digestible units. Several commercial brands are available in the form of powders, tablets, or capsules. The choice of enzyme and the dose must be determined for each individual. In general, weight gain and growth in infants and children is a sign of the effectiveness of the enzyme. The goal for adults is that they will maintain their normal weight.

Some vitamins must be dissolved in fatty material to pass through the intestinal wall. Even though digestion of fats is improved with pancreatic enzymes, children with cystic fibrosis require about twice the normal amount of vitamins A, D, and E daily. Supplements of vitamin K, another fat-soluble vitamin, are sometimes prescribed. There is no evidence that routine supplements of water-soluble vitamins, C and the B's, are warranted unless the child has a specific vitamin deficiency. If iron levels appear low, it might be necessary to add iron supplements to the diet.

Pancreatic insufficiency and the resulting intestinal malabsorption are the main reasons why children with cystic fibrosis need dietary counseling. In addition, chronic infection and increased expenditure of energy might result in the need for additional dietary supplements. Again, diets must be individualized after careful analysis of diet, energy requirements, and severity of malabsorption. Dietary supplements are usually high in calories and protein. Rich and tasty snacks such as milkshakes, puddings, and custards are not only useful, they are extremely popular! Diet supplementation is often necessary for children to maintain normal growth. Caloric intake might have to exceed the normal by 50 or 100%.

A small percentage of patients with cystic fibrosis have no apparent pancreatic deficiency or intestinal malabsorption. For them, treatment with pancreatic enzymes or fat-soluble vitamins may not be necessary. As discussed in greater detail in Chapter 7, recent research suggests that increased expenditure of energy is a fundamental expression of cystic fibrosis. For this reason, even patients with a normally functioning pancreas might require a high calorie and protein diet.

You may hear special dietary "breakthroughs" touted by the news media. A few years ago, several news organizations in the United States reported that the clinical problems in cystic fibrosis were due to a deficiency of the trace metal, selenium. Parents were encouraged to give their children massive doses of selenium, a cellular antioxidant. Tragically, several children died from toxic overdoses of selenium. In the last chapter, we discuss the arduous process of scientific investigation and give you some practical guidelines to evaluate so-called breakthroughs for cystic fibrosis.

Your child's physician is in the best position to advise you on "experimental" remedies. Have your doctor evaluate the new-found treatment before experimenting with it on your child.

Parents should be careful not to alter recommended levels of vitamin and diet supplements. If the doctor prescribes 800 International Units (IU) of vitamin D each day, don't think that 8,000 IU would be better. When it comes to medicines, more is not better.

Recent reports from clinical investigators suggest that patients with normal intestinal absorption may show a milder course of cystic fibrosis and a later onset of respiratory problems. Although not proven, aggressive nutritional management may result in overall benefit and improved function of the pulmonary system.

In summary, pancreatic enzymes play a crucial role in keeping patients with cystic fibrosis growing, healthy, and active. Your child's nutritional needs must be analyzed carefully and frequently by a dietician who, together with your child's doctor, will determine what is appropriate.

Meconium Ileus

Meconium, the excrement present in the intestinal tract of the fetus, is normally discharged at birth. The ileum is the lowest third of the three parts of the small intestine. (The duodenum is the upper third, the jejunum the middle third.) Failure to excrete meconium results in plugging of the ileum.

Meconium ileus, the medical term for the condition, probably develops because secretions of intestinal mucous glands are less soluble than normal and become difficult to excrete. In most cases, the plug can be removed by enemas containing substances that flush out the meconium. Surgery is required in some cases.

Meconium ileus occurs in 5 to 10% of children with cystic fibrosis. In a recent study of a large group of patients from Toronto, resarchers reported that 55% of children with cystic fibrosis born between 1958 and 1972 who had meconium ileus survived the first year of life, while 96% of the children born between 1973 and 1987 survived the first year. The condition has no impact on the course of the disease. Intestinal obstruction occurring later in life is called meconium ileus equivalent. In most cases, special enemas provide relief.

Other Problems of the Gastrointestinal Tract

The gastrointestinal tract includes all tissue extending from the mouth to the anus and organs associated with these tubes such as the liver and appendix. Problems with some of these structures and their functions result from pancreatic abnormalities, other problems directly from obstructive changes similar to those in the pancreas and lungs.

Stained Teeth

One unusual finding in some patients with cystic fibrosis is darkly stained teeth. The condition is not due to the disease itself but to its treatment. Antibiotics were introduced for the treatment of cystic fibrosis in the late 1940s. We now recognize that most individuals who used tetracyclines (a type of antibotic) extensively developed darkly stained teeth. Research showed that tetracyclines bind to developing bones and teeth, thus causing staining. Today physicians avoid prescribing tetracyclines for pregnant women and children under seven. Modern cosmetic dentistry can adequately treat the problem for patients who had received tetracyclines.

Diabetes mellitus

Diabetes mellitus is a complex condition in which sugar is not properly regulated by the body, resulting in increased sugar in the urine and blood. When a person swallows a concentrated sugar cocktail, it is possible to monitor the degree and speed with which the blood level returns to normal. This is called a glucose tolerance test. Impaired glucose tolerance (glucose intolerance) is present when blood levels of sugar are between normal and those considered diabetic. Both diabetes and glucose intolerance are common (about 40%) in people with cystic fibrosis, especially in older patients. Fortunately, the serious complications associated with ordinary diabetes are rare in patients with cystic fibrosis, and when necessary, the increased sugar levels can be controlled easily with insulin.

Rectal prolapse

Rectal prolapse, or protrusion of part of the rectum through the anus, occurs in about 20% of infants with cystic fibrosis before they are placed on pancreatic enzymes. It rarely occurs after five years of age. The condition is probably due to a combination of factors, including bulky feces, poor muscle tone, and increased abdominal pressure associated with a chronic cough. Avoiding constipation is the typical treatment. Surgery is rarely indicated.

Liver and Gall Bladder Complications

The liver and gall bladder, which functions as a storage sac for some liver products, are sometimes affected by cystic fibrosis. The abnormalities usually result from thick mucous secretions that obstruct tubes in these organs as they do in the pancreas. However, these problems are ordinarily not serious for individuals with cystic fibrosis. About 10% will develop gallstones, some of which will require surgical removal.

* * *

In the next segment from our Family Diary, Ben's father describes how "pills become part of the daily routine of life." The pills are pancreatic enzymes that allow Ben to properly digest food.

FAMILY DIARY

Many Pills

Medications are as much a part of life to a cystic fibrosis patient as food and water. Along with daily therapy, pills give children a chance to live fairly normal and active lives for many years. Just how many years varies considerably from patient to patient, but with new and better medications and treatments, people with cystic fibrosis are living longer all the time. That means hope, and to families who live with the disease, hope is everything.

Pills become part of the daily routine of life. As the years roll by, you tend to forget the amazement of strangers when they see such a healthy-looking kid swallowing pills by the fistful.

I'm reminded of that every time I head to our health maintenance organization (HMO) clinic on Ben's monthly drug run. We call in the order a few days ahead so the druggists have time to fill it. Most people waiting in line at the HMO pharmacy leave with a bottle or two, and tuck the month's supply of whatever into their purse or coat pocket. When a family with cystic fibrosis makes a stop—at least at our pharmacy—the month's supply doesn't fit through the pharmacy window. The druggist piles it into in a cardboard box and opens a side door to bring the load out to the waiting area.

I don't look up, but I imagine most people standing in line must have looks of disbelief. Who in the world could be THAT sick! I remember one time when Ben was standing in line with me. The druggist, a young woman, knew Ben's name quite well. She had typed his name on hundreds of jars and bottles, but she had never seen him in person.

"This is Ben?" she asked, unable to hide her surprise. "He looks . . . well, he looks so . . . so healthy." And he did, too.

Many of the pills are enzymes needed to digest food. His doctors also prescribe a variety of antibiotics, vitamins, and lung medications.

Once your child learns to swallow pills whole, the occasion is worth celebrating. It's as momentous as learning to walk or use the bathroom. For parents, you no longer have to empty the capsules, especially digestive enzymes, into applesauce to spoon feed them to your child.

Ben was swallowing whole capsules well before he started school. I think he was tiring of applesauce, too, since he'd eaten the stuff with every meal and snack since he was six weeks old. (Now that he's older and "off the sauce," he makes gagging sounds when we pass the applesauce section of the supermarket, especially when I pretend I'm going to buy a few jars.)

At first, Ben would swallow one or two of the enzymes at a crack; they're about the size of a cold capsule. Imagine my surprise when his day-care mother told me that Ben, probably showing off for his friends, swallowed six of the capsules at once. He was only four years old.

We keep little supplies of pills in many places: at grandma's, next to the cookies; at school, for lunch; in the car; at the neighbor's house; even in the backpack for picnics. If Ben eats without his enzymes, he develops a deluxe stomach ache and diarrhea. If he quits taking the pills, he wouldn't die the next day, or the next month, but he certainly would not be opening presents on his next birthday. We aren't tempted to skip medications. Ever.

Ben's classmates have grown accustomed to the pills and his meal-time routine, too. One day, when the teacher was a little slow bringing them to the lunchroom, they started to chant: "Ben needs his pills. Ben needs his pills. Don't forget the pills."

While his classmates realize Ben needs medications to remain healthy, they're more impressed with the fact that he's the fastest runner in third grade at St. James School and that he won the contest for holding his breath the longest underwater at day camp last summer.

Chapter 5
OTHER SYSTEMS

"She was my first baby. She was lovely
and the little salty taste tasted good. I didn't know that babies didn't
usually taste salty. My mother wondered about it, but we didn't do
anything until Amy started coughing a lot."

Cystic fibrosis affects nearly every organ of the body in some
way. Although the effects of the disease are most prominent
in the respiratory and digestive systems, other organs and
systems may also be impaired.

Sweat Glands

The primary function of sweat glands is to help regulate our
body temperature; 90% of heat loss occurs through our skin.
The glands also contribute to the excretion of 5 to 10% of our
metabolic wastes contained in the watery, salty, clear sweat.
On a daily basis, we produce anywhere from half a liter
(about a pint) to two or three liters. Evaporation of the fluid
helps regulate our body temperature. Sweat contains the
same substances—salts (sodium chloride), urea, and other
organic materials—as urine, but in a much more diluted concentration (Figure 14).

Here's how a normal sweat gland works: The deepest por-

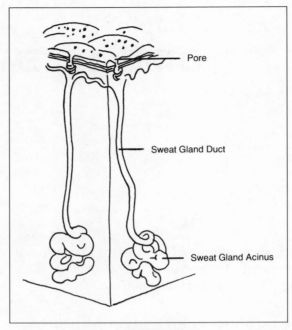

FIGURE 14

Sweat gland. Sweat formed in the acinus passes through tubes or ducts to the skin surface where it exits through pores. While moving through the ducts, much of the salt reenters the blood system. Because reentry of salt back into the body through walls of the ducts is greatly reduced in cystic fibrosis, the excreted sweat is salty.

tion of the sweat gland secretes a product containing water and small molecules from surrounding tissues. Some metabolic waste products are removed from the body in sweat. Other dissolved substances, such as sodium and chloride, are reabsorbed back into the body as the sweat moves toward the skin surface.

In sweat glands affected by cystic fibrosis, salt is not reabsorbed into the body properly, causing a higher concentration of salt and potassium in sweat. No relationship exists between the concentration of sweat salt and the severity of the disease. Abnormal concentrations of salt in sweat occurs in several other conditions, but these are easily distinguished from the lung and gastrointestinal problems associated with cystic fibrosis. Because the level of salt is the most constant laboratory finding in cystic fibrosis, sweat testing is routinely done to confirm the diagnosis. The abnormal sweat-gland function can have more critical consequences than a salty taste. Massive salt loss can lead to dehydration and heat prostration. If the patient is not cared for, shock can occur. In hot climates, during heavy exercise, or when a patient suffers a high fever, taking supplemental salt tablets or eating foods high in salt is necessary to prevent these complications. It may even be helpful to add salt to the patient's diet year-round. A patient's craving for salt should never be denied.

"I was 12 years old when the doctor told my parents and me that I would be sterile. I was a kid and knew that girls were different, but I didn't really think too much about it. When I got a little older and started finding out about sex, I became very depressed. Then I found out that being sterile wasn't the same at all as being unable to have sex. Things have turned out okay. I'm married. We've adopted a baby. We're doing okay. And my wife loves me."

Reproductive Systems

Because exocrine secretions are integral components of the body's reproductive system, cystic fibrosis can cause abnormalities in the sexual organs of both males and females. In general, the fundamental problem appears to be similar to the process in other organ systems—obstructions caused by thick, tenacious secretions with eventual damage to the obstructed structures.

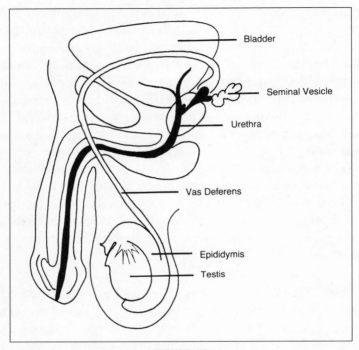

FIGURE 15

Male reproductive system. Sperm formed in the testes passes through a series of tubes. In most males with cystic fibrosis, mechanical obstruction prevents passage of sperm.

Male (Figure 15)

Sperm produced by numerous tubes in the testes are stored in the epididymis, a single large tube adjacent to each testis. Sperm pass from the epididymis through the vas deferens, the tube that is surgically tied and cut in a vasectomy. The vas deferens joins the urethra, a larger tube that connects the bladder to the outside of the body. Before the vas deferens joins the urethra, secretions from three glands (one of which is the seminal vesicle) generate the seminal fluid in which the sperm are suspended.

Approximately 98% of adult males with cystic fibrosis have

a mechanical obstruction that prevents the flow of sperm at the vas deferens, the epididymis, and the seminal vesicles. These obstructions apparently result from abnormal secretions into the affected tubes. The testes appear to show active but decreased production of sperm, which is probably related to the plugging. In effect, males with cystic fibrosis have a biological vasectomy. As with the surgical vasectomy, sexual potency is unaffected. Because the testes and sperm production are normal in males with cystic fibrosis, a bypass operation might someday allow males with the disease to become fertile. A semen analysis to determine the presence of sperm can be done when a male reaches sexual maturity.

The male sex organs and levels of male sex hormones are normal. Men experience normal sexual desires and are capable of normal sexual performance.

Female (Figure 16)

Each month, one or more eggs from a mature female are sloughed from the surface of the ovary and swept into one of the funnel-shaped Fallopian tubes where fertilization occurs. The Fallopian tubes descend to the upper corners of the pear-shaped uterus. The lower end of the uterus is formed by a firm muscular ring—the cervix—that extends a short distance into the vagina. The cervix normally produces large quantities of mucus.

Females with cystic fibrosis may have a delay in the onset of puberty, and their menstrual cycles may be irregular, depending on the individual's nutritional, pulmonary, and emotional status. However, the structure of the reproductive organs is normal, as is sexual desire. In mature females with cystic fibrosis, cervical secretions are excessive and thick. Plugging of the uterine opening by thick mucus acts as a barrier to sperm and may cause decreased fertility in women with cystic fibrosis. An estimated 85% of women in the general population are fertile, compared with about 20% or more of women with cystic fibrosis.

Women with cystic fibrosis can become pregnant, but they

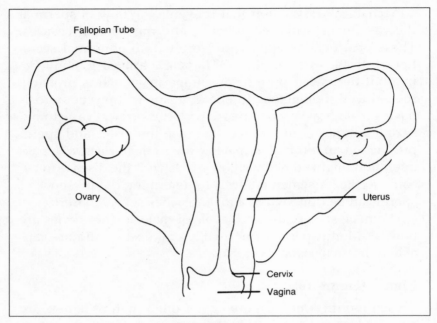

FIGURE 16
Female reproductive system. In mature females with cystic fibrosis, mucous lining the cervix (the entrance into the uterus or womb) is much thicker than normal and may make becoming pregnant more difficult.

have more spontaneous abortions, premature births, and stillbirths. These complications are probably related to maternal respiratory problems. Women who use oral contraceptives may experience cervical inflammation and occasional hepatitis-like symptoms.

Hundreds of pregnancies of women with cystic fibrosis have been reported. Because the pulmonary and cardiac demands of pregnancy may increase problems associated with cystic fibrosis, many cystic fibrosis centers advise women with the disease to avoid becoming pregnant. Women who do become pregnant should be followed by an obstetrician who is knowledgeable about cystic fibrosis.

Infants born to mothers with cystic fibrosis are not affected by their mothers' symptoms. It is possible that some drugs used in treatment may affect the development of the fetus. This should be carefully monitored. The risk of children born of mothers with cystic fibrosis having the disease is about 1 in 40, consistent with the risk from the estimated frequency of carriers in the general population.

Bones and Joints

The most obvious function of the skeleton is to give support and shape to the body. The skeleton protects underlying organs and works with a variety of joints and muscles to permit movement. A wide variety of problems related to bones and joints affects some people with cystic fibrosis. Scientists believe they result from problems of the respiratory or digestive systems.

Delayed Growth

As a group, children with cystic fibrosis are shorter than normal. However, numerous exceptions exist. The growth deficit becomes more marked in the pre-adolescent period because the natural "growth spurt" is often delayed in children with cystic fibrosis. However, many do eventually catch up and by adulthood the stature of some individuals with cystic fibrosis is in the normal range. Other children may not reach the stature of siblings or even parents. Respiratory dysfunction is believed to be responsible for delayed growth in some children; pancreatic deficiency, when treated with enzymes, should not by itself influence growth.

Clubbing

Abnormal growth of the tips of fingers and toes is probably due to enlargement of soft tissues under the nails. These areas are warm and tender. Clubbing is common in cystic fibrosis, and its frequency seems to increase with age. The cause is unknown, but it is clearly associated with lung disease. One theory is that substances produced in the body in response to lung infections affect these areas of the fingers and toes. There is no specific treatment for clubbing, but aggressive respiratory therapy may improve the condition.

Joint Pain

Joint pain may be a problem, particularly as individuals grow older. In a recent study, about 25% of adolescents and young adults with cystic fibrosis complained of pain in their knees, wrists, or ankles. The cause is unknown, but scientists suspect it is related to lung disease.

Kyphosis

About 25% of individuals with cystic fibrosis have an abnormal convex curvature of the spine when viewed from the side, a condition known as kyphosis. The condition worsens with age and relates to the barrel-shaped chest resulting from increased lung volume caused by obstructions.

* * *

As children with cystic fibrosis enter adolescence, they will have many questions about how the disease affects their bodies. In the next segment of our Family Diary, we see how Ben's father dealt with this sensitive issue.

FAMILY DIARY

A Father-to-Son Chat

"Dad, can we talk? I want to ask you about something?"

I knew by Ben's tone that the questions had been rolling around in his head for weeks. The time had come for another father-to-son chat about how cystic fibrosis affects daily living.

I was glad we had an open relationship; it makes it easier to have these kinds of talks.

'Sure, Ben, what's up?" I responded.

"So, am I always going to be so short?" he stammered.

The doctor had told me about the delayed development of children and adolescents with cystic fibrosis. What he didn't tell me—and couldn't—was how to always communicate this information sensitively to a precocious young boy.

Ben also knew what all the pamphlets and books said about growth. But the words don't always make sense to kids with cystic fibrosis, especially when they're lagging behind others in adolescent development. So I figured that Ben was wondering if CF had something to do with why he hadn't started changing like most of his friends.

"Hey, Ben, what makes you ask about that?"

"A basketball game. We were choosing teams at the playground after school and I was the last one picked again. It seems like I'm always the last one picked because I'm short."

My heart went out to him. Sports is so important for most boys, even when they have no illness. I was proud of Ben's determination to play. He worked hard at having fun. Like other kids his age, Ben's need for peer acceptance—to fit in with the gang at school—is strong. Besides the ability to compete in sports with his friends, I'm sure Ben was also becoming self-conscious about his appearance.

"Ben, I can only tell you what I know from the doctors. We've got to trust them on this one, because they've been right about the other things. Don't you think?"

"I guess so. Well what do they say? Will I always be short?"

"First of all, remember your size—height, weight, type of build—is a relative thing. You know, it becomes important when you start comparing yourself to other kids, especially to the biggest kids. You might be short compared to one person, but tall compared to another.

"Another thing to understand is the term median. It means average. When doctors talk about median height for boys with cystic fibrosis, they mean average. Some can be taller, others shorter."

Ben was listening, but I knew he was still looking for a more straightforward answer.

"Before we talk about you, let me throw out one more thing to think about. You're starting adolescence, and that's when bodies really change. You've seen how some of your classmates are growing, in some cases they're really shooting up. But I'll bet that some of them aren't growing as fast as others."

"I know that stuff, Dad, but I don't care about the others. What about me? What do the doctors say about me?"

"The doctors say you will grow, honest. Exactly when and how much, we don't know. That big growth spurt you're seeing in your friends is sometimes delayed for kids with cystic fibrosis. So, we don't know if you will always be the shortest kid on the team. In fact, you might end up being the tallest one in the class after you finish growing. Remember, those gene things we talked about, well height is determined by many genes in the body, genes that have nothing to do with cystic fibrosis."

Ben still looked troubled. He didn't have to like the situation, but now I think he understood it better because he managed a smile as he headed out the door with the basketball and a handful of cookies and enzymes.

"Where are you off to, guy?"

"I have to practice my shooting," he said. "Until I start all that growing, I'm going to work on having the best shot on the team."

Chapter 6
FAMILY LIFE

"**S**omewhere," *cried the young mother.*
"I'll find a doctor who can help."

"Why can't you accept the fact that Billy has cystic fibrosis," re-
torted her husband. "We've already been to experts in two states.
That means we only have 48 more to go."

"How can you give up on your child? Don't you love him?"

Chronic disease in children can lead to a host of social and
psychological problems for patients and their families. The
burden on the family may cause marital conflicts, limit social
life, distract attention from other children, and severely
drain financial resources.

Cystic fibrosis takes such a toll. Parents quickly realize that
time that would normally go toward one's spouse or family
fun activities may be consumed by daily treatments. But
there's a real reward for enduring the hardships—the chance
of a quality life for your child.

Many of the psychosocial issues associated with cystic fibrosis are commonly found with other congenital or chronic
diseases of childhood, such as sickle cell anemia, Down syndrome, cerebral palsy. Each disease, of course, generates its
own medical management problems, but the social and psychological dimensions are usually the same. In this chapter,
we'll see how they apply to cystic fibrosis.

Dialogue such as that contained in the quotation which

began this chapter is common among parents of children with chronic diseases or physical handicaps. One parent—it could be the mother or the father—accuses the other of failing to hope for a cure. Their spouse counters that it's time to accept reality. As mother and father blame each other for their child's predicament, more pressure is put on the marriage.

The family's role in the care and support of the child with cystic fibrosis begins in infancy and continues throughout her or his life. Health professionals guide the medical management, but only the family can provide emotional commitment and continuing care. Therefore, it is imperative that fathers and mothers learn to cope with their family crisis.

Family Adjustment

For the family to help their child, mothers and fathers, and sometimes siblings, must first accept the child's illness. It's natural to have strange and uncomfortable feelings and somewhat unrealistic expectations when you first learn that your child has a severe disease. Parents may feel shock. Even the most mature adult who claimed to be prepared for the worst news by asking thoughtful or insightful questions will be affected by the answers.

Once the initial shock wears off, the parent begins a ride on an emotional rollercoaster. This mixed bag of emotions is natural. Some days you feel in control—"Hey, I can handle this"—some days you'll lose it—"I hate this. CF care is all I do anymore." You will have periods of great optimism and times of deep despair. Part of this is the result of the indecisiveness on the part of doctors who, in many cases, cannot give you concrete answers about the child's prognosis.

The Grief Process

In 1969 psychiatrist Elisabeth Kubler-Ross published her classic study of death and dying. After counseling thousands of grieving people following the death of a loved one, she observed that the grieving process tends to fall into identifiable stages. Parents often experience the same kind of grief, although perhaps not as severe, when they learn that their child may have a severe illness or handicap.

The first reaction is usually one of denial. Parents may refuse to accept the diagnosis, and either ignore the physician's treatment plan or seek another opinion. The emotional turmoil takes a toll. Eventually, it must be vented, often in the form of anger. "Why didn't our pediatrician order a sweat test sooner?" The medical community is a frequent target of the enraged parent, and that's okay. Science doesn't have all the answers. Sometimes they misdiagnose. Often they just don't know. Anger can be healthy or harmful. It may be the first step toward useful action that will lead back to reality. It may persist and develop into guilt.

Most parents go through a unique phase that is not part of the traditional grief model. They believe that the child's disease may disappear, or perhaps a miracle will occur. They believe that medical science will achieve a breakthrough that will mean an end to cystic fibrosis for all children.

At the point of unrealistic hope, parents may place unrealistic expectations on their doctors. Some parents may bounce from one specialist to another. They begin to place too much hope on small improvements. They may turn to a minister or guru reputed to have healing powers. Of course, parents have the right to seek another opinion, or to pursue whatever therapeutic option they choose. But there comes a time when they must make a decision and get started with a medical treatment plan.

Parents who lose all hope are in a stage of acute grief, similar to a period of mourning. They consider their child's illness a punishment for their failures or misdeeds. This reaction is followed by a period of resignation or depression. It seems impossible to motivate themselves. During this time, they may even ignore appointments with the doctor. Sleep disorders and extreme fatigue may occur. These are symptoms of depression, and some form of professional counseling may be necessary.

After the anger and guilt, the grief and depression, parents reach a point of acceptance. It's the first step on the journey back to reality and the road to realistic hope. Energy and motivation return. And parents begin to enjoy the normal aspects of their child's life.

As the impact of the initial shock wears off, they learn that they still have much to be thankful for. Yes, they have lost their "perfect" child, but they learn to take pride in his or her achievements. They find that the loving bonds to their child are just as strong, or even stronger, than the bond between a mother or father and healthy children.

Help Is Available

Few of us have the strength to endure a traumatic emotional event without the help and understanding of others. Sometimes, we find this support in simple conversations with close friends or family members.

In many communities, parents have formed support groups where they meet to share feelings and provide a sounding board for questions and new ideas. How do you find such a group? Probably your best resource is your physician who knows hundreds of people in your situation or the local chapter of the Cystic Fibrosis Foundation.

Some parents need professional counseling to deal with their grief. You may feel more comfortable talking with your minister, priest, or rabbi. Licensed psychologists can be located in your local telephone directory. The county medical society may also put you in touch with a trained counselor.

A Coping Strategy

There is no easy path to mental, emotional, and spiritual well-being. Some families clearly cope better than others. Factors that might be important include a positive outlook on life, a belief that the family can make a difference in the child's illness, the quality of the marital relationship, honesty and openness within the family, and social and financial resources.

Here's a simple coping strategy that might work for you:

—Maintain a positive attitude. A father or mother who maintains an optimistic outlook on life instills a positive attitude in their child. A fatalistic attitude is clearly fatal in cystic fibrosis. Apathetic families produce apathetic children, and survival demands action and hard work to maintain good health.

—Trust your medical providers. Before chasing after a reputed cure touted by an obscure "expert," let your physician have a chance to counter the claim.

—In times of emotional crisis, consult a family counselor to resolve conflicts and improve communication. The counselor can be a member of the clergy, physician, friend, or professional psychologist.

—Become active in the local chapter of the Cystic Fibrosis Foundation. Share your experience with others who may be less knowledgeable about the illness.

—Interact with parents of other children with cystic fibrosis.

—Find role models for yourself and your child. Seek out young, successful adults with cystic fibrosis.

Home Care

Following confirmation of cystic fibrosis, the family must implement a program of "home care." The routine may be time-consuming, but it is necessary. Treatment is aimed primarily at keeping the lungs free from infection and maintaining normal gastrointestinal function through dietary supplements.

Small children may resist the daily regimen because it intrudes on their play time. They rebel at the loss of independence. Over time, they become cooperative, especially if the daily treatments become a natural part of the household schedule. It's best to approach home care matter-of-factly. If the procedure is hidden or performed secretly, the child will become embarrassed about his or her illness.

Most healthy brothers and sisters react to their chronically ill sibling in a positive manner, becoming protective. Of course, they may feel neglected at times. You can avoid such attitudes by having them share in the home-care routine.

Home life for a child with cystic fibrosis creates some special problems. The odor of stools might permeate the home, causing some family members to feel embarrassed in the presence of visitors. A persistent cough can be disruptive. Toilet training can be stressful because of the large bulky stools. Travel may be limited because of the threat of respiratory infections.

Hospitalization

From time to time, your child may be hospitalized because of acute flare-ups of disease symptoms such as lung infection or abdominal pain. Surgery, emergencies, or late terminal care may require prolonged hospital stays. How do you prepare your anxious child for the hospital experience? Here are some simple suggestions:

—For young children, separation from their parents is one of the most traumatic parts of the hospital experience. To ease the emotional burden on your child, request that you be allowed to share a room with him or her.

—Contact the hospital social worker assigned to the ward. He or she is your ally in dealing with the hospital rules and regulations, and can become an advocate in handling insurance companies.

—Frequent visits from friends and relatives also help reduce the feelings of separation and abandonment.

—Encourage small children to play out their anxieties with dolls. Of course, bring special toys, stuffed animals, and story books to the hospital.

—Some hospitals offer brochures or comic books describing the hospital experience to a young child. The hospital might also provide tours through children's wards before admission. (See the Section Resources at the back of the book for titles of several books on preparing children for hospitalization.)

—Adolescents are generally accustomed to the hospital routine, but they may feel uncomfortable if assigned to a pediatric ward. (Because cystic fibrosis was for so many years almost exclusively a disease of early childhood, most cystic fibrosis clinics and wards are ordinarily housed in the pediatric sections of hospitals.) Special arrangements may be made with the hospital to allow adolescents to share a room or to put them in a nearby ward.

Adolescence

Adolescence is a painful period because of the complex web of physical, sexual, and emotional changes occurring. Adolescents begin to strive for social and psychological independence. They assert their need for privacy and autonomy. It is a time for parents to begin letting go.

Adolescents seek approval from their peers. They are naturally concerned about the impression they make on the opposite sex. Most are future-oriented, defining their educational, vocational, and personal goals. Stereotypical adolescents can have other traits: erratic food habits, untidiness, and moodiness. To adults, adolescents seem to lack self-discipline.

A serious chronic disease superimposed on this dynamite period of life may seem overwhelming. Yet the mental state of most adolescents and young adults with cystic fibrosis is astonishingly healthy.

Physical growth and emotional maturation during adolescence may be slow. The usual anxiety over physical and sexual adequacy is intensified by the physical problems of cystic fibrosis. People with cystic fibrosis may be thinner and paler than others. The normal adolescent drive for independence is countered by medical and therapeutic dependency. They are caught in a constant tug-of-war between these opposing forces.

Manipulation of the adolescent's body by parents and therapists may cause embarrassment. Hospitalization emphasizes loss of privacy at a time when young people are becoming more modest. Adolescents may seek to minimize their daily therapeutic regimens, and they may resist hospitalization.

Special problems associated with cystic fibrosis can become especially aggravating to adolescents. The offensive odor of undigested fat in stools and the unpleasant loose cough and need to spit up phlegm cannot always be hidden. Neither can shortness, thinness, or paleness. Attempts at hiding the disease and forgoing treatment make things worse.

Education

Frequent absences from school may prevent academic excellence. Most teachers will offer special help or individual studies to compensate for the absences. Many school systems provide home-bound tutoring in cases of prolonged absences owing to illness.

Socialization

We can be heartened by the results of a study in the Neth-

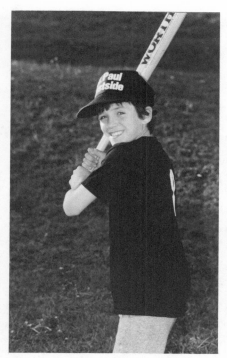

Left: Like so many with cystic fibrosis, Ben Winterer takes time each day for his therapy and then gets on with a busy and active life. He's fast, plays with spirit, and especially loves team sports like basketball and baseball.

Below: Any parent knows the feeling: "It's too quiet; that kid must be up to something." After digging around in his dad's closet, Ben came bounding down the stairs in clothing that—thanks to advances in CF care—he will one day grow into.

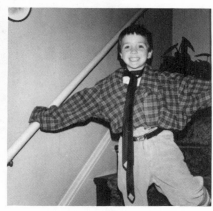

Below: Tired and content, Ben and his brother, Will, ran out of steam after a busy day and a ride home in the back seat of the family car.

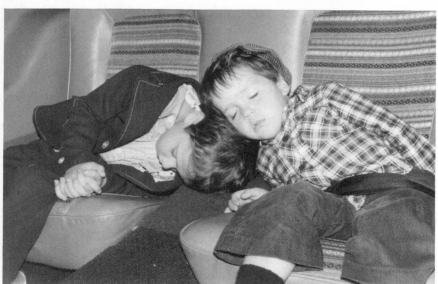

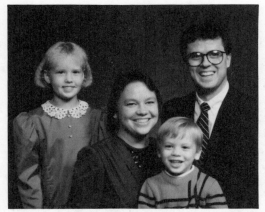

Mary Chalmers leads an active family life with husband, Chuck, daughter, Kara, and son, Nick. Both Mary and Chuck grew up in rural areas, and the family enjoys many outdoor activities like boating and hiking, Mary, who was diagnosed as having cystic fibrosis when an adult, is willing to talk with anyone who may have questions about CF.

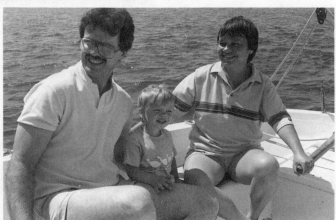

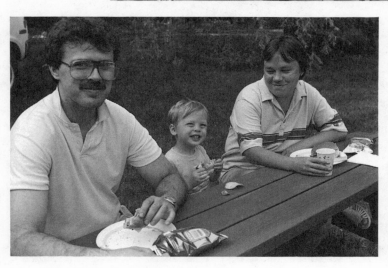

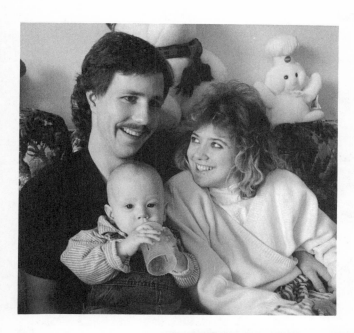

Stefani
McCulloch and
her husband,
Shawn, are kept
very busy with
their son,
Zachery. Stefani
also has a part-
time job. Photos:
Star Tribune,
Minneapolis.

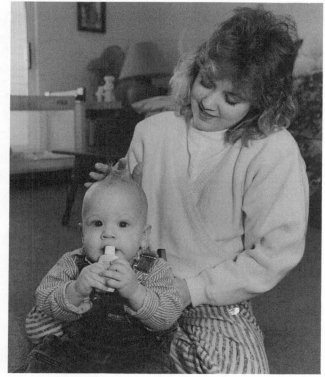

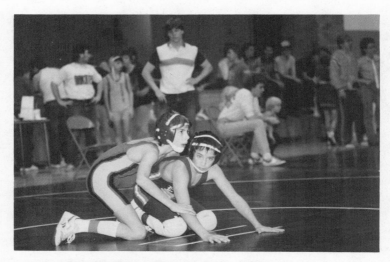

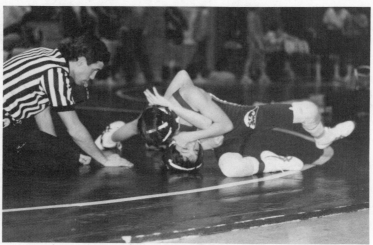

Brian Bakke enjoys many kinds of athletics, including wrestling.

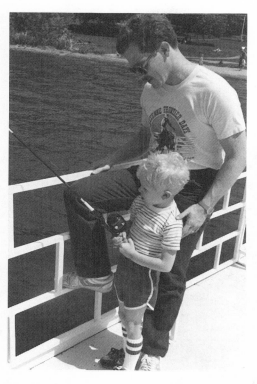

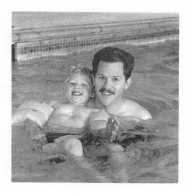

Cystic fibrosis isn't slowing down Andrew
Olson as he swims and fishes with his
dad, Larry.

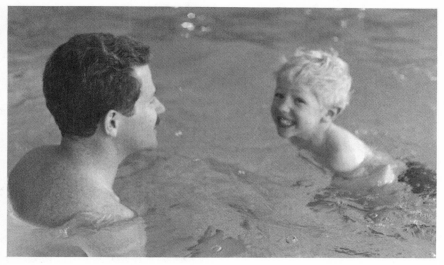

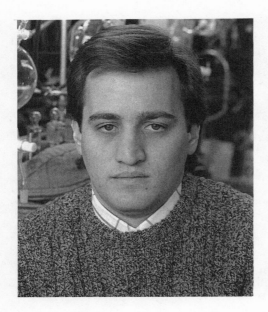

Tony DiMaio recently
completed his Ph.D. in
inorganic chemistry.

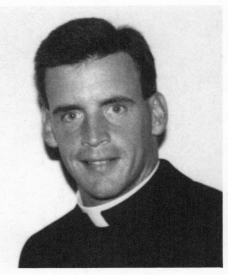

Gregory Tolaas, a priest at the
Campus Ministry, College of
St. Thomas, is from a family of
six children, four of whom
have cystic fibrosis.

erlands where adolescents with cystic fibrosis were compared with young people suffering severe asthma, healthy but small adolescents, and healthy individuals of normal size. Although 13- to 14-year-olds with cystic fibrosis showed a delay in "dating and mating" when compared with the other groups, they engaged in as many social activities outside the home as their healthy peers. There were no differences between the groups in the formation of ideals and the development of their own ideas about politics, religion, and ethics. The young people with cystic fibrosis were surprisingly optimistic about their future happiness despite possible setbacks.

Financial Problems

A chronic illness such as cystic fibrosis creates great financial burdens. Cost vary widely from patient to patient. In 1984 the estimated average cost per patient with cystic fibrosis was about $25,000 annually.

In many states in the United States, Crippled Children Services include cystic fibrosis as a disease eligible for assistance. Moreover, legislation has been passed in some states that provides financial help to people who are over 18 or 21. Major group medical insurance, paid entirely or in part by employers, is another common financial resource.

Medicaid payments are sometimes available for children who qualify for disability benefits. However, these benefits are only for families with very low incomes and few, if any, assets. While the program varies from state to state, very few patients with cystic fibrosis qualify for Medicaid benefits.

The Cystic Fibrosis Foundation sponsors a nationwide mail-order pharmacy so families can obtain drugs and dietary supplements at near-wholesale prices. (See Sources for the address and phone number of the pharmacy.) In some cases, major medical insurance covers drug costs. Many services, however, are not reimbursable.

Although health insurance plans show wide variability in coverage, they all have one thing in common: coverage ends at age 19 (or 23 if the individual is still in school) for those covered by their parents' policies. Adults with cystic fibrosis have a difficult time obtaining individual medical insurance. Many insurance plans are unwilling to cover an individual with a chronic illness. Group coverage is usually more complete with fewer limitations and less-stringent eligibility requirements.

"I'm 19 and I don't buy this stuff about a fatal disease. Everything is fatal. Some perfectly healthy football player died in a scrimmage. I wake up every day and eat and breathe and go to school and I'm going to do something with my life."

Death and Dying

"How long will our child live?"

The question looms over every clinic visit. Although rarely verbalized, parents naturally wonder if the latest infection or chronic cough may signify the beginning of the end.

Physicians cannot predict lifespan for children with cystic fibrosis. They can tell you the average life expectancy for all patients. They can also tell you what percentage of patients survive into adulthood. But it's impossible to forecast progression of disease in any patient.

Parents must be prepared to deal with the ultimate crisis in cystic fibrosis—the death of a child.

How do children view death?

A child's perception of death depends on age, social development, and attitudes of his or her parents. Infants and toddlers have no comprehension of death. About the age of 3, children begin to conceive of death as a temporary separation. To them, a dead person is on a journey or asleep. Between ages 5 and 9, children associate death with old age.

They believe death can somehow be avoided. A more realistic view of death begins to emerge at 10 to 12 years when children realize the permanence and inevitability of dying.

Children with life-threatening illnesses such as cystic fibrosis may have different perceptions, depending on their health history and what they've been told about their disease. Young children express fears of abandonment and bodily harm even when their concept of death is still vague. The most common questions of young children are: "Am I safe?" "Will somebody be with me to keep me from pain?" "Will I feel all right?" Older children, especially those who understand the medical problem, may show signs of depression. Children over 10 years of age become acutely aware of the seriousness of their illness and can experience grief and anxiety.

Children seem to pass through different stages during their illness. After children reach a point where they recognize themselves as being seriously ill, they progress to a time when they anticipate recovery. After a long period of illness, they come to believe that they have always been sick and lose hope of getting better. Finally, they develop an impending sense of death, often after observing the death of a fellow patient.

What can parents do to comfort their child? There is no perfect formula to manage this critical time. Most children respond better when they are told the truth about their condition. Many parents find these discussions emotionally unbearable and avoid the subject of death entirely. If a child appears ready to talk, then perhaps a physician or social worker can serve as the facilitator. Children should have the opportunity to question; they need answers in order to put their lives in order.

How do you know when a child is ready to discuss death? Some may be direct, while others use nonverbal cues such as play therapy or drawings.

Most terminally ill patients, including children, go through a stage of isolation. Their desire to be alone is a way of subconsciously separating themselves from loved ones. A child may become protective of parents and avoid discussion because they know it will hurt them. Although parents must be open, complete candor about the probable outcome is inadvisable.

How do parents cope with the loss of a child? Psychologists say the experience is the most stressful of all human traumatic events. Feelings that have been dormant or under control—guilt, blame, depression, impotence, frustration, and anger—may resurface and become exaggerated. Parents often feel a sense of failure.

Brothers and sisters may become anxious and confused. Some harbor a deep sense of guilt that they have survived. They often isolate themselves to reflect on their own mortality. Some resent the loss of their parents' attention and may even resent the dying child.

Every family must endure a period of grief and mourning. Family, friends, and clergy must form a support system during the time of anguish. Certainly, if the family in its grief and mourning becomes inconsolable and cannot function, psychosocial counseling should be considered.

* * *

The next installment of the Family Diary illustrates in a personal way how families pull together in the face of adversity.

FAMILY DIARY

No, He's Not from Outer Space. He's My Son

The weather forecast was calling for a beautiful Labor Day weekend, and we decided to squeeze in one last camping trip before the end of the summer. It wasn't going to be primitive camping, but as close as most cystic fibrosis families get to roughing it in the wild.

That's because people with cystic fibrosis can't wander too far from an electrical outlet. They need power for air compressors used to make a medicated mist. You might have seen pictures of kids with cystic fibrosis, with masks over their faces, in magazines or television commercials. They breathe the mist two or three times a day, for about 10 or 15 minutes, to help thin the sticky mucus in their lungs.

It was a busy weekend at the commercial campground; all the sites with electric hookups were long since taken. The camping routine for a cystic fibrosis family includes setting up the tent, shaking out the sleeping bags, cutting hot-dog sticks, starting a fire, and scouting out the handiest electric outlet.

We found two outlets, both located in the main campground building that housed an office, store, bar, bathrooms, and a video game room. The first outlet was in the shower and bathroom. But we had tried that before; it's not much fun. In most of the state campgrounds we've visited, the only available outlet was in the public bathroom. Besides the smell, you have to deal with 15 minutes of stares and questions from well-meaning but curious bathroom patrons. So you stand there, as other people use the toilet, shave, brush their teeth, and spit in the sink . . . and wonder if the camping experience is worth all that.

The other available outlet that Saturday night seemed more promising. It was located off in a corner of the video game room. With all those dingdinging, rat-a-tat-tat, kabloom, and revving motor sounds coming from the video games, who'd notice the hum of an air compressor and a little masked kid with a swirl of mist around his head.

Not so. Unfortunately, a few minutes after we hooked up the mask and turned on the compressor, kids began flocking into the game room. Some were camping there like us, but others were from the surrounding farming area. We were in THEIR Saturday night hangout.

There were 25 or 30 of them in the room; it was just about elbow-to-elbow. We soon realized Ben wasn't just tucked in an out-of-the-way corner. He was the star attraction. A few kids started plugging quarters into the machines, but most

formed a semicircle around us and stared. These weren't
subtle, sideway glances. We were used to those. These were
full-bore stares. Nobody said anything; there were no questions. Just stares. Here was a kid who looked like one of the
outer-space creatures in the video games. He came complete with smoke and a hissing sound. Ben was on display,
and it hurt; a heavy load for a seven-year-old.

We were far from our comfortable living room, where "doing the mist" is a quiet, family routine; something to do while
reading or watching a favorite television show. But this was
frustrating and embarrassing.

"Dad, how much more time?" he asked quietly. What he
really meant was: "Dad, let's get outa here!"

I looked at the electronic timer. "We're about half done,
Ben."

"Okay," he said, and that was all. He just sat there and
looked down at his new Velcro sneakers.

I knew Ben was hurting. I wanted to jump up and yell at
those kids to stop staring. But it would have called even more
attention to my son. You try to live your life so that cystic fibrosis isn't a big deal. You take the pills and do the therapy so you
stay healthy and out of the hospital. You do your cystic fibrosis
chores each day, then you put it aside and live like any other
family.

I looked down at the timer. He still had several minutes to
go. "All done, Ben, let's go back to camp," I lied. He took off
the mask and helped coil up the cord and air tube. We
grabbed the compressor and broke through the crowd. "Zoo
time's over, kids," I thought to myself. "Go back to your video
machines."

Ben held my hand as we walked into the warm summer
evening. The friendly smell of campfires was a nice change
from the medicated mist smell, a not-so-distant cousin to
smoldering rubber. Soon we'd be at our own campfire, with
friends, where 45 minutes of hard pounding on Ben's chest to
knock loose the mucus wouldn't be a big deal—just part of
cystic fibrosis life. Ben's older brother, Will (bless his endearing

patience), would wait till the pounding was finished so we could all roast marshmallows together.

"Dad," Ben said as we walked back to camp, "let's do the mist real early tomorrow morning. Okay? Before those kids come down there."

"Sounds like a good idea to me," I said. "Hey, Ben?"

"What, dad?"

"I sure was proud of you tonight."

Chapter 7
HORIZONS OF RESEARCH

"**M**y son with cystic fibrosis is nearly 11 now and he's doing just great. People who are kind and well-meaning sometimes ask if he'll outgrow the disease. I tell them no, of course, but it's nice to leave them with some hope. I tell them that for almost every year since he's been born, the average length of life for patients with CF has increased another year because they have found better ways of treating the symptoms. Sure he's got CF, but my son is thriving and healthy and, I hope, will continue to be.

"You've got to be realistic and I'm not expecting it to happen tomorrow, but if research comes up with some solution or cure for the basic CF defect, I want my son to have his health so he can take full advantage of the discovery. It's something we talk about every now and then . . . like when he has to come in early from playing ball to do therapy, even though he feels fine."

How can we gauge our efforts at conquering cystic fibrosis?

One barometer of success is mean life span. CF is no longer solely a disease of children. Before the advent of antibiotics and digestive enzymes, the majority of children died in infancy. The most common causes of death were lung and heart failure, and an inability to digest food, which leads to starvation. In 1955 only 50% of children with cystic fibrosis lived to four years of age. The mean life span began to increase dramatically beginning in the early 1960s for several reasons: centralization of care at specialized cystic fibrosis

treatment centers, intensive chest physiotherapy, and powerful antibiotics.

Today, the mean life span is about 27 years. But many individuals live much longer. In 1980, 45 patients had survived
to age 40, five to age 50, and a few have lived into the sixth
generation of life.

Extending the life span of children would not have been
possible without basic research into the disease. And science
has made quantum leaps in understanding the disease process while developing better methods of diagnosis and treatment. One way of charting medical advances is by the number of studies recorded in medical journals. In 1960, 75
medical or scientific papers dealing with cystic fibrosis were
published in reputable medical journals. That figure doubled
by 1970 and today more than 300 papers are published each
year. The range of research is vast, encompassing social and
psychological topics (what are the most effective means of
coping?), clinical management (does active exercise help or
hinder? which antibiotic is most effective?), and the applica-
tion of techniques of modern molecular biology (what is the
basic genetic defect leading to the disease?).

Theoretically, cystic fibrosis should be easy to understand.
A double dose of a gene produces a gene product that leads
to manifestations of the disease. This is certainly a more simple condition than cancer, in which cells multiply out of control in many different ways, or Down syndrome, in which
many extra genes are found in cells. The problem with cystic
fibrosis is that we still have not identified the abnormal gene
product and its function. Once the abnormal protein is un-
covered, much of the puzzle will fall into place. Until then,
scientists will continue to accumulate pieces of information
here and there. Even minor discoveries can directly affect
and improve a patient's condition.

In this chapter, we shall describe how medical research is
done and mention several avenues of that research. We cannot review all current research into cystic fibrosis. That
would require several volumes. Rather, we have chosen a

few areas that have potentially important implications for patients and families.

Locating the Cystic Fibrosis Gene

In 1985 researchers in England, Canada, and the United States showed conclusively that the gene responsible for cystic fibrosis was on chromosome 7. Geneticists have found sites or "markers" on chromosome 7 that appear very close to the cystic fibrosis gene. The "markers" can play an important role in diagnosing cystic fibrosis, even in an unborn child.

To explain the role of markers, let's examine a family with a child named Peggy who has cystic fibrosis. We know that both of her parents have the responsible gene on one of their number 7 chromosomes and its normal counterpart on the other number 7 chromosome.

The process of identifying those markers begins with an ordinary blood sample. Blood is obtained from each parent. Then, the blood cell's DNA is examined for marker A, which is known to be close to the cystic fibrosis gene on chromosome number 7. Marker A can be in one of two forms—"A1" or "A2"—and each form is easy to identify. Because marker A and the cystic fibrosis gene (or its normal counterpart) are very close to each other, they are usually passed together from parents to children. In other words, they are not separated by the normal shuffling of genes when eggs and sperm are made.

In examining Peggy's DNA, we learn that she carries marker A1 on both of her number 7 chromosomes. But each of her parents has marker A1 *and* A2. We already knew that Peggy has the cystic fibrosis gene on both number 7 chromosomes while each parent has the cystic fibrosis gene on one number 7 chromosome and its normal alternative on the other. The question is: which A marker is linked to the cystic fibrosis gene, and which one is linked to the normal gene in

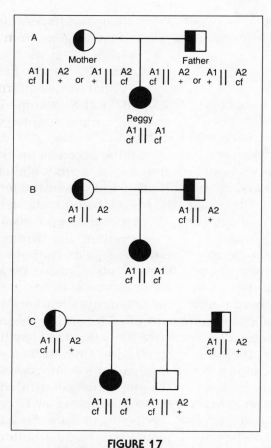

FIGURE 17

Prenatal diagnosis of cystic fibrosis using DNA. ○ = female, □ = male, ◐ or ◨ = known carrier for cystic fibrosis, ● = female with cystic fibrosis. (See text for explanation.)

Peggy's parents? In Figure 17, we show symbols for Peggy and her parents. Under each symbol is the cystic fibrosis and marker A status of each.

Remember, we knew from DNA testing that Peggy was A1/A1. Since the A site on chromosome 7 is very close to the cystic fibrosis gene, information at the A site and the cystic fibrosis site sort together during egg and sperm formation. Since Peggy received the cystic fibrosis gene from both parents and she has only the A1 marker, the cystic fibrosis gene must be linked to A1 and not A2 in this family. Each of Peggy's parents has a chromosome 7 that carries information for A1 and cystic fibrosis, and another chromosome 7 that carries information for A2 and the normal counterpart of the cystic fibrosis gene (Figure 17b).

Let's assume that Peggy's mother becomes pregnant again and she and her husband choose to learn whether the new baby would have cystic fibrosis. Cells from the fetus can be obtained from the amniotic fluid bathing the fetus in the mother's uterus. These cells can be tested for markers in the manner explained above. By studying the chromosomes of these cells, the baby's sex is determined. The baby has one X and one Y chromosome—a boy—symbolized by a □ in the pedigree in Figure 17c.

The analysis revealed that the fetus's markers are A1/A2. The baby will not have cystic fibrosis because the presence of the A2 marker in this family means that the baby has at least one normal gene. As we learned in Chapter 1, a single normal gene (even if the counterpart is a cystic fibrosis gene) is sufficient for normal functioning. However, the fetus is a carrier for cystic fibrosis, just as his parents are. To confirm the prenatal diagnosis, the new baby will have a sweat test.

Obviously, the technique is useful only if both of Peggy's parents have both forms of the marker. For example, if her father was A1/cystic fibrosis and A1/normal on his two number 7 chromosomes, there would be no way to determine which number 7 was associated with the cystic fibrosis gene.

However, there are now a dozen markers that are very close to the cystic fibrosis gene. The chances that this technique will be valid for prenatal diagnosis in a family where cystic fibrosis has already occurred is greater than 97%. For the test to be useful, DNA from both parents and the child with cystic fibrosis must be available.

A more recently developed method for obtaining DNA from a fetus uses cells from the chorion, a second membrane which encloses the fetus and has minute projections called villi. Chorionic villus cells are obtained by inserting a flexible catheter through the vagina and cervix, and, with the guidance of ultrasound, moving the tube to the fetus. An approach through the abdomen, also with ultrasound guidance, may be at least as safe. The great advantage of chorionic villus sample (CVS) over amniocentesis is that DNA can be obtained between 8 and 10 weeks after conception—two months earlier than amniocentesis. Terminating a pregnancy during the first trimester is simpler than during the second.

What are the practical uses of DNA screening?

In countries where therapeutic abortion is legal, parents may decide to terminate the pregnancy if a screening test confirms cystic fibrosis. Prenatal diagnosis has other uses. It will relieve the anxiety of many parents because 75% of the fetuses will have no evidence of the disorder. Another benefit of prenatal testing for cystic fibrosis is the possibility of early diagnosis. Although not proven it is generally believed that the earlier treatment begins, the better the course of the disease. Therefore, newborns identified as having cystic fibrosis (with confirmation by a sweat test shortly after birth) will begin receiving prophylactic treatment almost immediately, thus staving off infections and complications.

Identifying the Cystic Fibrosis Gene

In September 1989 three extremely important research papers co-authored by twenty-five scientists from Toronto and Michigan appeared in one issue of the magazine *Science*. In these articles, the gene responsible for cystic fibrosis was identified. The investigators made use of the very new technology of "reverse genetics." Basic genetic defects are usually determined by tracing back from an abnormal protein to a gene. However, in the case of cystic fibrosis, the abnormal protein was not (and still is not) known. Using the extremely powerful techniques of molecular biology, these researchers were able to completely characterize the DNA that is responsible for cystic fibrosis. The DNA is arranged in triplets, which code for a protein composed of 1,480 amino acids. In 68% of chromosomes carrying the cystic fibrosis gene, the DNA triplet coding for amino acid #508 is missing. This triplet was present in 100% of normal chromosomes. Other alterations in the same gene account for the other cases. The remaining changes in DNA responsible for cystic fibrosis have not yet been identified but may be by the time you read this book. The researchers predicted that at least seven additional DNA changes will account for the remaining 32% of cases. They also discovered that there are two genetically distinct types of cystic fibrosis: about 85% of patients have digestive problems resulting from a malfunctioning pancreas and about 15% have few or no digestive problems. Most of the patients with digestive problems are missing amino acid #508.

This extraordinary work makes it possible to identify approximately 70% of carriers in the general North American population. Based on their analysis, the scientists predict that they will be able to identify 57% of white couples who are at risk of having a child with cystic fibrosis. That proportion does not include Jewish couples of Central European origin. In that ethnic group the cystic fibrosis mutation that has been identified causes the disease only 30% of the time. Other studies have shown that the discovered defect is responsible for about 70% of cases in the United Kingdom but less than 50% in Spain and Italy.

And these investigators have suggested that their findings may provide for the development of improved means of treatment. While this is the hope and may be achievable, we must remember that the basic defect in sickle-cell anemia was discovered in 1948 and we still do not have a suitable treatment for it.

It may seem odd that the gene responsible for cystic fibrosis and the amino acid sequence that it directs is known completely through this monumental work, and yet, as the authors acknowledge, the basic biochemical defect remains unknown. One way of understanding this apparent contradiction is to think of finding a key. Using the bumps and valleys on the edge of the key, a locksmith could reconstruct the patterns of tumblers in a lock in which the key could work. We have found the key (the gene) and the lock it can open (the amino acid sequence) but we don't know where the original lock (the one that counts) is. That is the problem as of this writing. To completely understand the basic defect in cystic fibrosis it will be necessary to identify the abnormal protein and to determine what its role in the disease is. Enormous progress has been made and the prospects for a complete understanding of cystic fibrosis are promising.

Salt Transport

In Chapter 5 we discussed the sweat gland abnormalities in cystic fibrosis. In recent years, scientists discovered that an important abnormality in cystic fibrosis is the regulation of cell membrane channels through which chloride enters and exits cells.

Work from several laboratories has shown that abnormal transport of chloride across sweat glands, nasal and tracheal cells occurs in cystic fibrosis. The electrical properties of these cells are altered, which may lead to physical abnormalities in mucus. As explained earlier, mucous obstructions underlie many of the problems found in cystic fibrosis.

Chloride moves in and out of cells through specific channels in cell membranes. These chloride channels function abnormally in cystic fibrosis. Scientists recently demonstrated that the number and structure of the channels are normal, indicating that the regulation of these channels by other substances in the cell must be the problem. Research is now underway to learn more about regulation of chloride channels and how it malfunctions in cystic fibrosis.

Understanding the role of chloride may lead to a unifying hypothesis about cystic fibrosis. The discovery may also open up a new avenue for treatment.

Energy Metabolism in Cystic Fibrosis

As mentioned in Chapter 5, the delayed growth and generalized gauntness in many individuals with cystic fibrosis has been attributed to lung disease. This may be so, but recent studies from research centers in Great Britain and Australia indicate that increased energy metabolism—a hypermetabolic state—occurs in patients with cystic fibrosis. Hypermetabolism may contribute to depressed height and weight, More important, hypermetabolism may be an expression of the fundamental cellular abnormality in cystic fibrosis.

In the British study, 23 subjects (12 males and 11 females) were chosen randomly from patients at a cystic fibrosis outpatient clinic. None of the children was acutely ill, 20 of the 23 were receiving pancreatic enzyme replacement therapy, and 8 of the 23 were receiving nebulized antibiotics for chronic pulmonary *Pseudomonas* infections. A control group consisted of 21 boys and 21 girls who were healthy siblings of patients with asthma.

To test the expenditure of energy while resting, subjects lay on a bed with an acrylic hood with a loose-fitting collar placed over their heads and shoulders. During a preliminary rest period of 30 minutes and a 15-minute test period, the children listened to music or watched TV. Room air was gently sucked through the hood, and oxygen and carbon dioxide concentrations were determined during the test period.

In the subjects with cystic fibrosis, energy expenditure was significantly elevated, suggesting that the rate of metabolism increased in these individuals. Apparently, the difference between patients and controls was independent of age, sex, or body size.

Simultaneously with publication of this study, an independent research group in Australia reported similar findings using other methods. In this study, 9 infants with cystic fibrosis ranging in age from 0.7 to 2.0 years, were tested. None had lung disease or was receiving antibiotics. All 9 were receiving physiotherapy, and 7 of them were also receiving pancreatic enzyme and dietary supplements, 2 were underweight and 2 had had lung infections. The control group included 16 healthy infants who were matched for age and weight with the cystic fibrosis group.

Tests were carried out over 12 days. The infants were fed water that had low concentrations of radioactive oxygen and hydrogen. Urine was collected with cotton pads placed in diapers, and total energy expenditure was calculated from the proportion of radioactive and non-radioactive oxygen and hydrogen eliminated in the urine.

The researchers found that energy expenditure was increased by about 25 percent in subjects with cystic fibrosis. This difference was unrelated to weight, lung disease, or pancreatic insufficiency. The scientists concluded that the basic cellular defect in cystic fibrosis may be one of altered energy balance through an energy-consuming abnormality.

We find these results extremely interesting in light of our own work at the University of Minnesota Health Sciences Center. Nearly 10 years before these clinical studies were published, we showed that cells from subjects with cystic fibrosis and parent carriers consumed more oxygen than did controls. Subsequent experiments suggested to us that the basic defect in the disease is related to an increased energy metabolism at the cellular level.

The relationship between findings of hypermetabolism and chloride transport has not yet been unraveled, but the question is being pursued actively by many scientists throughout the world.

Evaluating a New Treatment

How should parents react to news reports on the latest "breakthrough" in cystic fibrosis research?

Knowing how legitimate researchers perform studies may help you evaluate news of the latest drug, vitamin supplement, or medical device. The following "case study" was conducted by a group of researchers at Harvard University to determine the effectiveness of anti-inflammatory drugs such as cortisone on the course of the disease. The questions could be applied to most studies.

QUESTION: How many patients were in the study? (That's important to know because the fewer the patients, the less chance there is to show a significant finding.)

The Harvard researchers identified 45 patients with cystic fibrosis ranging in age from 1 to 12 years. They accepted only those with mild to moderate lung disease since they thought these children would be a better group to test the effect of the drug than were children who already suffered irreversible lung damage.

QUESTION: How did the researchers ensure objectivity?

The researchers randomly assigned (like flipping a coin) children to either a treatment group or a placebo (a "sugar pill," not real medication) group. The drug and placebo looked and tasted the same. To ensure there was no bias on the part of the research team, they were not told which children received the drug and which the placebo. This procedure is called a "double-blind" study.

QUESTION: Why are placebos necessary? Why not simply give patients the new drug?

Researchers proceed on the assumption that they don't know if a test compound will make a difference. There's always the possibility that the drug might be harmful. In this study, the side-effects of anti-inflammatory drugs were already documented. Study subjects were informed of the risks of participating, as well as the potential benefit.

QUESTION: How was the study designed?

The children were examined and given laboratory tests at the beginning of the study and then periodically (monthly or every six months, depending on the test) during the next four years. The following information was obtained: pulmonary function, liver function, blood-cell counts, chest X-rays, sputum and throat cultures, and height and weight.

QUESTION: Was there a "control" group used for comparisons?

A third group of 69 patients with cystic fibrosis who chose not to participate in the study were followed during the same period of time to see how their health changed.

QUESTION: What did the study prove?

At the end of the four-year study, significantly more children in the placebo and control groups were hospitalized for flare-ups of pulmonary problems than children receiving cortisone. Statisticians used a mathematical formula to show that the possibility the differences observed were due to chance and not the drug were less than one in 1,000. The treatment group scored significantly better in some pulmonary tests, such as vital capacity. However, there was no difference in other tests, including chest X-rays. And researchers noted there was no difference in the incidence of infection with *Pseudomonas*. The average height and weight of children in the treatment group were significantly greater at the study's end. The placebo and control groups were similar.

QUESTION: Did the drug cause any side-effects?

The researchers reported children treated with cortisone experienced no harmful side-effects.

QUESTION: What conclusions did the researchers draw from their study?

In their words: "Our findings suggest a role for anti-inflammatory agents in the therapy of CF pulmonary disease, but this conclusion must be tempered by the small size of the study population and the short observation period. A group with little structural lung disease was chosen for the study because these patients would be more likely to respond to anti-inflammatory therapy. Thus, we cannot yet recommend the addition of corticosteroids to conventional therapy of all or even most patients with CF, but the findings do provide the basis for further study of the long-term benefits and potential complications of anti-inflammatory therapy in this disorder."

QUESTION: Does this study mean that every child with cystic fibrosis should take steroids?

No. Although the study was conducted by reputable scientists and closely monitored by outside experts, the findings still must be confirmed by other investigators. Such studies are currently underway.

QUESTION: Why does research move so slowly?

From the perspective of patients and families, the process of science proceeds at a snail's pace. But there must be safeguards to prevent errors that could ultimately produce inaccurate results and harmful outcomes.

QUESTION: How do I learn about progress in cystic fibrosis research?

Although the news media often report major developments in this disease, newspapers and television are often poor sources of information because they omit important details. Probably the single best source of a balanced interpretation of new research is the Cystic Fibrosis Foundation (the foundation's address and phone number are listed in the Resources section at the back of the book.)

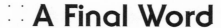

A Final Word

The last excerpt from the Family Diary ends this book where it began, with the involvement of family in treatment of cystic fibrosis.

"I was getting sick and tired of the whole thing. Ben was having lung problems again, and it seemed like that's all we did anymore . . . treatments, treatments, treatments. When I collapsed into bed late that night, I felt something under the pillow. I turned on the light and cried while I read this note:

Thank you DaD
for going thro all
this troble to
make me A live

"He's only eight; I didn't know he even thought about the stuff I did."

GLOSSARY

Some words defined here do not occur in the text but are relevant to cystic fibrosis.

Acini. Small sac-like clusters at the tips of branched tubes in glands; major gland products are made in acini.

Acute. Severe and of relatively short duration.

Acute respiratory failure. Occurs when the exchange of gases between the circulating blood and the atmosphere is impaired suddenly and severely; depressed oxygen levels in the body affect cellular metabolism of all organs and can cause damage in minutes; requires emergency treatment.

Aerosol. A fine mist containing liquid or solid particles of medicine for inhalation.

Albumin. Any of several simple proteins found in blood serum, egg whites, and many tissues.

Allele. One of the possible forms of a gene.

Alveoli. Tiny air sacs of the lung at the end of bronchioles, where exchange of oxygen and carbon dioxide between the lung and blood takes place.

Amino acids. Twenty small compounds that are the subunits of proteins.

Amniocentesis. Passage of a needle through the abdominal wall into the uterus to obtain amniotic fluid and cells from the fetus.

Anemia. A reduction below normal in the oxygen-carrying capacity of blood.

Antenatal. Before birth.

Antibiotics. Any of various substances produced by fungi, bacteria, and other organisms or made synthetically that inhibit the growth of or destroy bacteria and other organisms.

A-P diameter. The anterior-posterior (front to back) measurement of the chest, often increased in cystic fibrosis.

Apnea. The temporary absence of breathing.

Aspermia. Failure of formation or emission of sperm.

Aspirate. To remove liquids or gases from a space by suction.

Asthma. Reversible obstruction of airways not owing to any other disease.

Atelectasis. A shrunken and airless state of part or all of the lung.

Atrophy. Shrinking of tissues or organs.

Autosome. Any chromosome that is not a sex (X or Y) chromosome.

Azotorrhea. Excessive loss of nitrogen in the feces reflecting decreased absorption of protein because of pancreatic deficiency.

Bacteria. Any of numerous single-celled micro-organisms having a wide range of biochemical and often pathological properties.

Barrel chest. Increase in front-to-back diameter of the chest secondary to chronic respiratory disease.

Bile (acid). A fluid made in the liver, stored in the gall bladder, and discharged into the small intestine; aids digestion, chiefly of fats.

Biopsy. The removal and examination of tissue as an aid to medical diagnosis.

Bleb. A small blister.

Bronchial drainage (chest physical therapy, postural drainage). The assisted movement of mucus from the lungs through a combination of chest percussion and appropriate positioning of the subject.

Bronchiectasis. Chronic widening of bronchial tubes with cough and secondary infection.

Bronchioles. Thin-walled extensions of bronchi connecting them to lung alveoli.

Bronchiolitis. Inflammation of the finer branches of the branched bronchial tree associated with respiratory distress and wheezing.

Bronchitis. Acute or chronic inflammation (infectious or chemical) of the lining of the trachea and its two large branches, the bronchi.

Bronchodilator. Several classes of drugs that dilate (open wider) bronchial tubes. They operate through relaxing muscles surrounding the tubes and by interfering with cell systems that constrict the respiratory tubes.

Bronchoscopy. A technique that permits the physician to directly visualize the lungs through a tube passed down the throat.

Bronchus. One of the two major branches of the trachea leading to the lungs.

Caloric intake. An estimate of available biochemical energy derived from the diet.

Carbohydrates. Any of a group of chemical substances, including sugars and starches, that contain carbon, hydrogen, and oxygen; a major source of body energy.

Cardiac enlargement. Enlargement of a heart chamber owing to abnormal overwork of the heart (see COR PULMONALE).

Carrier (heterozygote). A normal person who possesses one copy of a gene that in a double dose would result in an observable characteristic.

Cervix. The lower and narrow end of the uterus that extends into the vagina. Covered by mucous-producing epithelial cells.

Cholecystitis. Acute or chronic inflammation (reaction to injury) of the gall bladder.

Chromosome. Threadlike structures in nuclei of most cells; they carry genes.

Chronic. Persisting over a long period of time.

Cilia. Tiny hair-like structures attached to the outer edges of some cells that are capable of rhythmic movements.

Cirrhosis. A chronic disease of the liver with progressive destruction and regeneration of liver cells and scarring.

Clubbing. An enlargement of tips of fingers and toes; the cause is unknown but is associated with chronic lung disease.

Congenital. A condition present at birth.

Cor pulmonale. Enlargement of the right ventricle of the heart (which pumps blood from the heart back to the lungs); the most common cause is chronic obstructive lung disease.

Cough. A sudden, noisy expulsion of air from the lungs, a natural mechanism for clearing the respiratory tract; a cough in which sputum is removed from the lungs is a productive cough.

Cyanosis. A bluish discoloration of the skin owing to inadequate blood oxygen.

Cystic. Pertaining to a sac or sacs lined by a membrane that frequently contains fluid or semi-solid material.

Dehydration. Excessive loss of water from the body, which may result from loss of body salts and diarrhea.

Diabetes mellitus. A chronic disease often with deficient pancreatic insulin production, inability to metabolize carbohydrates resulting in increased blood and urinary sugar.

Diaphragm. Large muscular partition separating abdominal and chest cavities; the most important breathing muscle.

Digestion. Bodily process by which food is broken down into particles small enough to be transported from the digestive tract into the blood stream.

Digestive system. The various tubes, organs, and accessory glands involved in digestion.

DNA (deoxyribonucleic acid). The component of chromosomes that carries genetic information.

Dominant trait. A genetic trait that is expressed in heterozygotes for the gene.

Ducts. Tubular passages through which secretions are carried.

Duodenum. The first portion of the small intestine extending from the lower end of the stomach to the jejunum, the second part of the small intestine.

Dysfunction. Disordered or impaired function of a bodily system or organ.

Dyspnea. Difficult or labored breathing often associated with heart or lung disease.

Eccrine. Secreting externally; exocrine.

Edema. An excessive accumulation of fluid between cells of a tissue.

Emphysema. Enlargement or inflation of air sacs in the lung secondary to obstruction; results in labored breathing and increased susceptibility to infection.

Empyema. Accumulation of pus in a body cavity such as the chest.

Endocrine glands. Any of several ductless glands which secrete hormones directly into the blood system, e.g., thyroid or adrenal gland.

Enzyme. Any of numerous proteins produced by living organisms that function as biochemical catalysts (increase rates of chemical reactions without themselves being changed); they are highly specific and function in very small quantities.

Enzyme replacement. Treatment of an inborn error of metabolism by introducing a missing or defective enzyme; generally not yet successful.

Epididymis. Long tube along the side and back of the testes in which sperm are stored.

Esophageal varices. Abnormally dilated and twisted blood vessels (varices) around the esophagus; may be due to increased resistance in the liver to blood flow secondary to cirrhosis; characterized by gastrointestinal blood.

Exocrine glands. A gland that secretes its product through ducts or tubes onto internal or external body surfaces.

Expectorants. Products that promote expulsion of materials, particularly mucus, from the lungs.

Fats. Composed of carbon, hydrogen, and oxygen as are carbohydrates but with much less oxygen; important as biological fuels and as structural components of cells.

Fatty infiltration, liver. Abnormal accumulation of fat in liver cells; a common response of the liver to injury.

Fibroblasts. Cells of supporting tissues of the body such as those beneath the surface of the skin; relatively readily grown in culture and useful in biomedical research.

Fibrosis. Replacement of the essential elements of an organ by scar tissue.

Focal biliary cirrhosis. Obstruction of bile ducts in the liver by secretory plugs similar to those found in the pancreas. Scarring is spotty (focal).

Gall bladder. Pear-shaped reservoir near the liver for bile made in the liver.

Gall stones. Solid concretions formed from insoluble cholesterol in bile, may cause abdominal pain.

Gamete. A germ cell containing half the number of chromosomes of a body cell; mature sperm or ovum.

Gene. The fundamental unit of heredity; a slight change in a gene can result in a slight change in its product—a protein—with wide-ranging consequences or a slight change may make no apparent difference.

Gene pool. All the genes present at a particular chromosomal location in the population.

Genetic code. There are four DNA bases; different combinations of three (triplets) code for the 20 amino acids.

Genetic counseling. Information about transmission of the gene for cystic fibrosis and other genetic conditions, risks of occurrence, and reproductive planning.

Genotype. The genetic constitution of an individual or the alleles present at one locus (particular site on a chromosome).

Glucose. One of several simple sugars which in combination form the large carbohydrates that we eat; breakdown of glucose in cells is a major energy source for cell function.

Glucose tolerance. Ability of the body through the action of insulin and other metabolic regulators to maintain a normal blood glucose concentration after ingestion of a glucose cocktail.

Glycoproteins. Any of a class of proteins that have associated carbohydrates; the chief constituents of mucus are glycoproteins.

Heart failure. The clinical condition resulting from inability of the heart muscle to pump enough blood to tissues of the body.

Heat stroke. Sudden and severe attack with dry skin, headache, dizziness, and cramps; may result from excessive loss of sodium and chloride and water in hot weather or during fever.

Hematemesis. Vomiting of blood (see ESOPHAGEAL VARICES).

Hemophilus influenzae. A species of bacteria important in causing a wide range of human disease, particularly respiratory disease.

Hemoptysis. Coughing up of blood as a result of respiratory tract bleeding.

Heterozygote. An individual who has two different forms of a gene (alleles) at a given place (locus) on a pair of chromosomes (see CARRIER).

Heterozygote advantage. In some environments, a person heterozygous for a particular gene may have a survival advantage over those with identical genes on a chromosome pair.

Histology. The microscopic study of the structure of tissues.

Homozygote. An individual who has identical genes at a given place (locus) on a pair of chromosomes.

Hypochloremia. A decrease in blood chloride levels.

Hyponatremia. A decrease in blood sodium levels always associated with water loss (see HEAT STROKE).

Hypoproteinemia. Abnormal decrease in blood protein concentration owing to defective digestion and absorption of protein from the diet because of pancreatic enzyme deficiency.

Hypoprothrombinemia. Prothrombin is converted to thrombin in blood plasma in one of the stages of blood clotting; Vitamin K controls formation of several clotting factors including prothrombin. Vitamin K deficiency secondary to pancreatic deficiency can result in hypoprothrombinemia with hemorrhage.

Hypoxia. Abnormally low oxygen concentration.

Iatrogenic. Resulting from a physician's actions.

Ileum. The third portion of the small intestine extending from the jejunum to the beginning of the large intestine.

Immunity. The state of being resistant to a disease, especially an infectious disease.

Inborn error of metabolism. A genetically determined biochemical disorder that has pathological consequences.

Intussusception. An infolding of one part of the intestine into an adjacent section.

Iontophoresis. The introduction by means of an electrical current of substances into body tissues; used, for example, to induce sweating in the skin sweat test.

Jaundice. Yellowish discoloration of tissues and bodily fluids caused by blockage of bile from the liver to the intestine.

Jejunum. The second of three segments of the small intestine.

Kyphosis. Abnormal curvature of the spine with rearward convexity.

Lavage. The irrigation or washing out of an organ or part of an organ.

Lethal equivalent. A gene, which if present in two doses in an individual, is lethal; it is estimated that each individual carries three to five lethal equivalents.

Lipids. Any of numerous fats and fatlike materials insoluble in water. Important for energy and for cell structure; digestion of them is impaired in cystic fibrosis.

Liver. A large gland in the upper abdomen on the right side; produces bile and functions in the metabolism of carbohydrates, fats, proteins, minerals, and vitamins.

Lobe. A portion of an organ.

Lobectomy. Surgical removal of a portion (lobe) of an organ.

Locus. The position of a gene on a chromosome; different forms of a gene are often found at the same locus.

Malabsorption. Impaired absorption of nutrients from the small intestine into the body.

Malnutrition. Any disorder of nutrition that may result from inappropriate dietary intake or, in the case of cystic fibrosis, inappropriate processing of nutrients.

Meconium ileus. Intestinal obstruction (ileus) by fetal intestinal contents (meconium) that are normally excreted at birth.

Meconium ileus equivalent. Meconium ileus (intestinal obstruction) seen in older patients.

Metabolism. Complex physical and chemical processes by which foods are broken down for use in the body.

Mist tents. Tents with high mist for overnight sleeping to improve lung function; no longer in general use.

Molecular genetics. The study of the structure and function of genetic systems in terms of the chemistry and physics of their molecular constituents.

Morbidity. The condition of being diseased; the ratio of sick to well persons.

Mortality. The condition of being subject to death; the death rate.

Mucolytic. Destroying or dissolving mucus.

Mucus. Thick suspension of glycoprotein, water, cells, and salts secreted as protective lubricant coatings by some glands.

Mucous membrane. Membranes lining all bodily channels that communicate with the air.

Mutation. A permanent, heritable change in the genetic material.

Myocardium. Heart muscle.

Nasal obstruction. Partial or complete blockage of nasal passages by nasal polyps.

Nasal polyps. Benign growths arising from nasal linings by enlargement and blockage of mucous glands in the lining; almost always associated with sinusitis.

Nebulizer. Converts a liquid into a fine spray for inhalation.

Neonate. Newly born infant.

Ovum. An egg cell.

Pancreas. Long, soft irregularly shaped gland lying behind the stomach that secretes pancreatic juice containing digestive enzymes into the duodenum; also produces insulin which is sent directly into the blood system.

Pancreatic enzymes. Enzymes that break down proteins, fats, carbohydrates, and nucleic acids.

Pancreatitis. Inflammation of the pancreas.

Parenteral. Taken into the body other than through the digestive tract, e.g., intravenously or intramuscularly.

Pathogen. Any agent that causes disease; a bacterium, a chemical, an abnormal gene.

Pathognomonic. Something so specific to a disease that a diagnosis can be based on it; meconium ileus and elevated sweat chloride are almost pathognomonic for cystic fibrosis.

Pedigree. In medical genetics, a diagram representing a family history and showing affected individuals.

Percussion. Striking a part of the body with short sharp blows as an aid in diagnosing the condition of the parts below by the sounds made.

Phenotype. The total physical, chemical and psychological nature of an individual produced by genes and environment; in a more narrow sense, the expression in the individual of a particular gene.

Phlegm. Stringy, thick mucus secreted by glands lining the respiratory tract.

Physical therapy. The treatment of disease or injury by mechanical means such as exercise, massage, postural drainage.

Pilocarpine. A drug that stimulates sweat glands to secrete; applied by iontophoresis before testing for sweat salt concentration.

Pneumonectomy. The surgical removal of lung tissue.

Pneumonia. An acute inflammation or infection of all or parts of the lung.

Pneumothorax. Free air in the chest outside the lungs.

Portal hypertension. Increased blood pressure in the liver associated with increased circulatory resistance in the liver to blood flow; may lead to esophageal varices and gastric bleeding.

Postural drainage. See BRONCHIAL DRAINAGE.

Prognosis. A prediction of the probable outcome of a disease or likelihood of recovery; in medical genetics, the probability of recurrence of the disease or condition in another member of the family.

Prophylaxis. The prevention of disease; preventive treatment.

Protein hydrolates. The breakdown products of proteins after their digestion by pancreatic enzymes in the small intestine or artificially.

Proteins. Any of a group of large nitrogen-containing compounds made up of amino acids; occur in all living tissue and are essential for growth, repair, and function.

Pseudomonas aeruginosa. One of several species of *Pseudomonas*; as cystic fibrosis progresses, it is the most frequent isolate from sputum; it is more difficult to eradicate than other respiratory bacteria in cystic fibrosis.

Psychosocial. Behavioral and social consequences of a medical problem and their management.

Pulmonary. Pertaining to the lungs.

Pulmonary edema. Accumulation of fluid between cells in the lung; a consequence of heart failure.

Pulmonary function tests. Include numerous, varied, and sophisticated ways to evaluate normal and abnormal working of the lung and its parts.

Pulmonary hypertension. Increased blood pressure in the lung's circulation; associated with decreased oxygen and structural changes in blood vessels; can lead to heart failure.

Pulmonary insufficiency (or respiratory failure). Occurs when the exchange of air between the circulating blood and the atmosphere is deficient; the effect of decreased oxygen in arteries and tissues depends on degree; if severe, irreversible damage to cells can occur; if moderate and prolonged, it can lead to pulmonary hypertension and heart failure.

Pulmonary osteoarthropathy. See CLUBBING.

Purulent. Consisting of or containing pus.

Reabsorption, salts. All secretions contain salts and other small substances and water that must be returned to the body before the secretions finally leave the body; failure of reabsorption leads to deficiency.

Recessive trait. A trait that is expressed only in homozygotes for a particular gene.

Rectal Prolapse. Protrusion of the rectum through the anus.

Recurrence risk. The probability that a genetic disorder present in one or more members of a family will recur in another member of the family.

Residual lung volume. The amount of air remaining in the lungs after maximal expiration.

Respiration. The act of inhaling and exhaling; the metabolic process whereby an organism uses oxygen and releases carbon dioxide and other products of oxidation.

Respiratory failure. Impairment of exchange of oxygen and carbon dioxide between air and blood.

Respiratory system. The organs and tubes associated with the exchange of gases between the organism and the environment.

Rhinitis. Inflammation of the nasal mucous membranes.

RNA (ribonucleic acid). A nucleic acid with similarities to DNA that functions in the translation of the genetic code to protein synthesis.

Salivary glands. Glands that secrete saliva into the mouth; there are three pairs of large glands and hundreds of minor glands.

Scoliosis. Abnormal side-to-side curvature of the spine.

Seminal vesicle. Paired structures in the male situated above the prostate gland; a major source of seminal fluid in which sperm are suspended.

Sinusitis. Inflammation of the linings of air-filled cavities (sinuses) of head bones which communicate with the nostrils.

Splenomegaly. Enlargement of the spleen; among many causes are chronic infection and cirrhosis of the liver.

Sputum. Expectorated matter including saliva, substances from the respiratory tract, and foreign material.

Staphylococcus aureus. A common bacterial organism associated with lung infection in cystic fibrosis.

Steatorrhea. Excessive loss of fats in the feces.

Sterility. The state of being free of microorganisms; the inability to produce offspring.

Sweat electrolytes. The small, electrically charged molecules excreted with sweat, e.g., sodium or chloride.

Sweat test. The determination of the concentration of chloride or sodium in sweat; the most reliable diagnostic test for cystic fibrosis.

Thoracic cage. The bony structure made up of ribs, breastbone, and backbone that encloses and protects the heart and lungs.

Tissue. An aggregation of structurally and functionally similar cells.

Trachea. The tube that carries air into the bronchi.

Triglycerides. The storage form of fatty acids in cells that yields high energy when broken down by cells.

Vas deferens. Part of the male reproductive system involved in the ejaculation of sperm; in cystic fibrosis, it is usually obstructed.

Ventricle. Two lower chambers of the heart that pump blood throughout the body or to the lung.

Viscous. Having a relatively high resistance to flow.

Vital capacity. The maximum volume of air that can be expired slowly and completely after a full inspiration. A valuable measurement of lung function.

Vitamin A. Found in fish, liver, oils, egg yolk, dairy products, and green leafy vegetables; involved in vision and health of skin and membranes.

Vitamin D. Found in fish liver oils, butter, and egg yolk; also produced in the body in response to sunlight; necessary for normal bones and teeth.

Vitamin E. Found in vegetable oil, wheat germ, leafy vegetables, egg yolk, and pod vegetables. Functions as an antioxidant in cells and in cell membrane stability.

Vitamin K. Found in leafy vegetables, pork liver, vegetables oils. Necessary for blood clotting.

Vitamins, fat soluble. Vitamins such as A, D, E, and K which are absorbed through the intestinal wall only when in solution in fats.

Volvulus. Obstruction caused by abnormal intestinal twisting.

X-linked genes. Genes situated on the X chromosome.

THE CYSTIC FIBROSIS CARE TEAM

Children with cystic fibrosis should be examined, treated, and followed at specialty clinics staffed by teams of experienced health-care professionals. These centers, which are sponsored by the Cystic Fibrosis Foundation, apply a "team" or "multidisciplinary" approach to meeting your child's special needs. Here is a brief description of the different members of the cystic fibrosis medical team:

Consultant. A physician who provides expertise in addition to that possessed by team members. Your child's doctor may request a consultation from a specialist in, for example, endocrine diseases (perhaps to check blood sugar or insulin levels) or infectious diseases.

Dietician. A professional who applies principles of nutrition to your child's diet and provides special diets at the physician's request.

Fellow. A physician who, following a specialty residency, studies a medical sub-specialty such as pediatric pulmonology. Fellows work closely in a master-apprentice relationship with the specialist. Under supervision, fellows help perform many specialized procedures such as bronchoscopy.

Genetic counselor. A professional trained to provide information to patients or relatives at risk for a disorder that may have a genetic basis. The counselor discusses consequences of the disorder, the probability of developing and/or transmitting it, and ways in which it can be prevented in future pregnancies.

Licensed practical nurse (LPN). A nurse with a two-year degree who works under the supervision of physicians and registered nurses (RNs). The LPN performs many of the same tasks as the RN, but does not have the same level of training.

Medical technologist. A person trained in laboratory techniques who carries out a broad range of complex chemical, microscopic, and bacteriological laboratory procedures to help identify and control disease.

Neonatologist. A pediatrician who specializes in the care of newborns.

Nurse Practitioner (clinician). A registered nurse (RN) with additional formal education and experience that makes possible an expanded role in health care. Activities may include taking health histories, performing physical examinations, ordering and interpreting diagnostic tests, and, in consultation with the physician, planning treatment.

Nursing assistant (aide). A person who provides patient care that, although not requiring highly technical skills, is basic to the comfort and well-being of the patient.

Pediatrician. A physician who specializes in diagnosis and treatment of individuals who are usually under the age of 18.

Physical therapist. An allied health professional who, upon a physician's referral, evaluates and treats physically impaired individuals in areas such as musculoskeletal, cardiovascular, or respiratory functions.

Pulmonologist. A physician specially trained in the diagnosis and treatment of lung and chest diseases.

Radiologist. A physician who specializes in the use and interpretation of x-rays for diagnosis.

Registered nurse (RN). A nurse who received training in delivery of services such as determining body temperature, pulse rate, blood pressure, and other vital signs. The RN prepares the patient for examination and assists the physician. A nurse may administer medications and other treatments under direction of the physician.

Resident. A physician in an educational program to become a specialist.

Respiratory therapist. An allied health specialist trained in the treatment and management of patients with serious lung and heart disease. Working under the direction of the physician, a respiratory therapist has more responsibility for patient care, teaching, and supervision than does the respiratory technician.

Respiratory therapy technician. Often supervised by the respiratory therapist, the technician carries out noncritical respiratory treatments.

Social worker. A professional who focuses on the psychosocial problems of the ill patient and the patient's family including locating sources of financial assistance and coordinating services.

RESOURCES

There are more than 120 cystic fibrosis centers in the United States, 31 in Canada, and 25 in England. Staffs of these centers include physicians, respiratory and physical therapists, nurses, psychologists, and social workers who have expertise in the diagnosis and treatment of cystic fibrosis.

For locations of cystic fibrosis care centers, contact

in the United States:

> Cystic Fibrosis Foundation
> 6931 Arlington Road
> Bethesda, Maryland 20814
> (301) 951-4422 or toll-free, 1-800-FIGHT CF

> Cystic Fibrosis Foundation Pharmacy
> 11420 Rockville Pike
> Suite 10
> Rockville, Maryland 20852
> 1-800-541-4959

in Canada:

> Canadian Cystic Fibrosis Foundation
> 2221 Yonge Street
> Suite 601
> Toronto, Ontario, Canada M4S 2B4
> (416) 485-9149

and in England:

Cystic Fibrosis Trust
Alexandra House
5 Blyth Road
Bromley, Kent
United Kingdom BR1 3RS
(011-44-1-464-7211

Besides identifying the cystic fibrosis care center nearest you, these foundations are the health organizations dedicated to finding new and better treatments and a cure for cystic fibrosis. They should be contacted if you want to obtain information on the latest research findings and treatment advances in cystic fibrosis.

USEFUL BOOKS

More technical discussions of cystic fibrosis

Goodfellow, P. *Cystic Fibrosis*. Oxford University Press, Oxford, 1989.

Lloyd-Still, J.D. *Textbook of Cystic Fibrosis*. John Wright Inc. Boston, 1983.

Orenstein, D.M. *Cystic Fibrosis*. Raven Press, New York, 1989.

Taussig, L.M. *Cystic Fibrosis*. Thieme-Stratton Inc., New York, 1984.

About coping

Gots, R. and Kartman, A. *The People's Hospital Book*. Avon, New York 1981.

Kushner, H. *When Bad Things Happen to Good People*. Schocken Books, New York, 1981.

Mitchell, J. *Taking on the World*. Harcourt Brace Jovanovich, New York, 1982.

For children

Howe, J. and Warshaw, M. *The Hospital Book.* Crown Publishers Inc., New York, 1981.

Livingston, C. and Ciliotta, C. *Why Am I Going to the Hospital?* Lyle Stuart, Secaucus, N.J., 1981.

INDEX

INDEX

Compiled by Eileen Quam
and Theresa Wolner

BURTON L. SHAPIRO, Ph.D., professor of oral science and laboratory medicine and pathology and member of the Institute of Human Genetics at the University of Minnesota Health Science Center, has been on the faculty of the University of Minnesota since 1966. He has served on the board of directors of the Minnesota Chapter of the Cystic Fibrosis Foundation. Widely published, Shapiro contributes to such journals as *Nature, Science*, the *American Journal of Human Genetics*, the *American Journal of Medical Genetics*, *Lancet*, and *Life Sciences*.

RALPH C. HEUSSNER, Jr., has been a medical writer at the University of Minnesota since 1980. Previously, he was a reporter and editor at *The Atlanta Journal & Constitution*. He is the co-author of *Herpes Diseases and Your Health* (University of Minnesota Press, 1984) and *Warning! The Media May Be Harmful to Your Health! A Consumer's Guide to Medical News and Advertising* (Andrews & McMeel, 1988).